Gorilla and the Bird

Gorilla and the Bird

a memoir of madness and a mother's love

ZACK McDERMOTT

Little, Brown and Company
New York Boston London

Copyright © 2017 by Zack McDermott

Little, Brown and Company
Hachette Book Group
1290 Avenue of the Americas, New York, NY 10104
littlebrown.com

First edition: September 2017

Little, Brown and Company is a division of Hachette Book Group, Inc. The Little, Brown name and logo are trademarks of Hachette Book Group, Inc.

The publisher is not responsible for websites (or their content) that are not owned by the publisher.

The Hachette Speakers Bureau provides a wide range of authors for speaking events. To find out more, go to hachettespeakersbureau.com or call (866) 376-6591.

ISBN 978-0-316-31514-2
LCCN 2017936279

10 9 8 7 6 5 4 3 2 1

LSC-C

Book design by Marie Mundaca

Printed in the United States of America

For Granny, the Bird's Bird

AUTHOR'S NOTE

This is a true story, and I have done my best to ensure accuracy in its telling. As my memory is sometimes fallible, dialogue is approximate. In cases where the events described took place when I was too young to understand what was happening around me, I have relied on my mother, the Bird, to fill in the gaps. The names and identifying details of some individuals have been changed.

Gorilla and the Bird

PROLOGUE

GRANNY HATES THE PIGS to this day. If she's in a friendly mood, she'll call them "the fuzz," but never just "the police" or even "cops." Most often, it's "the pigs." "Zachariah, look out the window. Is that the pigs?" She'll say that in the same voice she uses when she says "Look, there's a cardinal in my bird feeder" — nonchalant, lacking any malice. It's purely observational: *There's a bird. There's the pigs.* One night in 1978 the pigs beat her son Edward senseless on her front lawn while she watched.

My uncle was sitting in the cab of Pa's truck, stoned out of his mind on PCP, when the cops showed up. First two cars, then three, then six. When they started pounding on the driver's side window, Pa told them they didn't need to do that. "Let me talk to my son and I'll get him out of the truck." He was told to "stay on the porch, sir." Then to "stay on the fucking porch, sir." Soon he realized he should not have told the cops that Edward was strong, that he didn't know for sure what he'd taken, and that his son wasn't in his right mind. They interpreted that as *Please beat my son's ass because he is definitely going to try to beat yours.*

Edward came out swinging once they got the door open, so high on dust that he didn't know he didn't have a chance. They beat him and kept beating him with their billy clubs while he flailed and resisted. Then they beat him after he quit flailing. Then they beat him after they cuffed him. Then they maced him. Then they kept beating him.

My mother, the Bird, knew why her parents' house was lit up in blue and red before she got close enough to see the cop cars covering the front lawn. *Edward*. It couldn't be anything but Edward. Pa was on the porch, three cops forming a moat around him. He was howling, crying so loud she heard him before she got out of the car. Edward was in the backseat of one of the cruisers. The blood matted his hair down and caked his cheeks. His face was starting to swell, but he'd look much worse in the morning. He was smiling.

Granny couldn't talk for several hours, and what she saw that day would haunt her forever. Edward, shackled and maced and bathed in police lights, getting bludgeoned by six men with wooden batons. Her husband screaming and cussing and crying and begging. Sirens ringing in her ears. Black baton hitting skull with the same pop as bat hitting baseball. The beating was brutal enough to have killed him, for sure. At what point could she be certain that it hadn't? Never. And if the beating hadn't finished him off, the PCP might still have had something to say.

The Sunday after Thanksgiving 1982, a few months before I was born, my schizophrenic uncle Eddie suffered his last overdose on angel dust. He was airlifted to Kansas City with a heart aneurysm. The procedure they used on him was new enough that his case was later chronicled in medical textbooks. The doctors gave him less than a 30 percent chance of making it through the surgery.

His body survived, but in many ways, that was the end of his life. After the airlift, Granny and Pa stayed with Edward in the Kansas City ICU until just before Christmas. Granny prayed the rosary; Pa drank whiskey.

This last overdose, combined with his already severe and untreated mental illness, erased any lingering hope that he might someday be able to live anything approximating a "normal" life. The schiz and the addiction—proverbial chicken and egg—had swallowed the man. He was twenty-six years old.

Granny and Pa didn't want him institutionalized, but he couldn't live on his own either. He could barely control his own body. Given his age, Granny and Pa couldn't just tell him he had to live at home. In an attempt to regain guardianship, they went to court. Things didn't go according to plan. The judge lifted their burden of care entirely—they were denied guardianship. Edward was ordered to enter a state mental institution in Topeka.

On the day the men from the mental hospital came to pick up Edward, my mom went into labor with me. His last day on the outside was my first.

CHAPTER 1

I WALKED OUT OF my apartment on the corner of St. Marks and Avenue A that afternoon and I knew we were rolling. I knew the people on the sidewalk were actors. They resembled the normal East Village lot, but they were archetypes: the skaters were all wearing DC Shoes and expensive skinny Levi's; the construction workers' boots were too worn, their accents too Brooklyn thick; and what kind of girl wears Louboutins in this neighborhood? Even the homeless people were a little too attractive, and when I looked closely, I could tell their face tattoos were actually professional makeup jobs.

It made sense. I'd spent the whole summer doing stand-up and writing a TV pilot with The Producer, a new friend with major connections whom I'd met at an open mic. He'd assured me that he had access to anyone we wanted to work with in Hollywood, and earlier in the week we'd met with an MTV producer who'd expressed interest. Now, a few days later, I found myself in a real-life audition. The Producer's approach was genius: just let me do what I do, interact with the common folk, and get it all on film. It was up to me to make the show work. All the production assistants were doubling as extras, their foot traffic directing me from one scene to the next.

The herd steered me toward Tompkins Square Park at the end of my block. I couldn't believe how well they'd cast Generic Old Man on Park Bench. In comedy, it's the little details and cameos that separate good from great, after all. I knew the old man should be my first mark, so I approached him immediately. I said hello. He looked nervous but returned the greeting. I grabbed his bike with the intention of taking it for a few laps. "No!" he shouted as he yanked it away. The old man had some chops. Figuring our scene was up, I sprinted east toward the dog park and hurdled the fence. Before popping back out at the end of the dog run, I dropped down on all fours to gallop with the pack.

Any minor doubts that we were shooting were eliminated when Daniel Day-Lewis power-walked across the basketball court. He was dressed in full *Gangs of New York* regalia: top hat, coat, and long waxed moustache. The Producer knew he was my favorite actor and must have convinced him to make a cameo just for the hell of it. Day-Lewis, a legendary practical joker, must have done it for free because we certainly couldn't afford him. This little inside joke was The Producer's way of telling me "Yes, this is happening. Trust your instincts. Make comedy gold."

On the corner of Houston and First Avenue, knowing the streets had been closed for me and the cars were piloted by professional drivers, I sprinted across the intersection, narrowly avoiding several taxis as they braked and swerved. The ratio of yellow cabs to regular commuters was about 70/30, closely approximating the real split in New York but slightly inflated on the taxi end since it made for a good visual.

I trespassed into one of the Lower East Side's public housing buildings. Like many of the places I'd been that day, the inside of the projects looked so authentic that it had to be artificial, a caricature of itself. *Do people really leave the doors to their apartments open while their shitty televisions blare into the hall? Is Mami really cooking up some Puerto Rican food on that two-burner hot plate? What's next, a guy in a dirty wifebeater drinking malt liquor and screaming on the fire escape?* These must be establishing shots, designed to show the audience that, yes, we were actually shooting in New York, the non-*Friends* version. I walked out an emergency exit and set off the alarm.

Down the block from the projects was a park with a mini AstroTurf soccer field. Rec league players passed the ball around; their game was about to kick off. Perfect! I had played soccer in college. I sprinted onto the field, ushered the keeper aside, and started yelling at the players.

"Have one, ya wee pisser!" I shouted in a Scottish accent.

The forwards obliged and started shooting. No one could beat me. My movements were effortless. I could read the trajectory of the ball and anticipate its dips and arcs as soon as it left the shooter's foot — like a Major League Baseball hitter who can spot a curveball as it leaves the pitcher's hand. I batted eight or nine shots away before relinquishing the goal back to the team's keeper. He looked too impressed to be pissed.

"That's how it's done, son." I sauntered out of the box.

"Get the fuck off the field!"

I looked around, trying to figure out who they were yelling at.

"Get the fuck off the field!"

"Me?"

"Yes, you!"

Jealous. With your goddamn shin guards on like you're playing in the World Cup. I pulled my shorts down past my butt and started jogging laps around the field, bare-assed. Occasionally I'd turn at midfield and sprint across the centerline. I could run for days.

"Get the fuck off the field!"

I continued to run, both on and around the soccer field, throughout the entire first half before noticing that many of the players were facsimiles of guys I'd played with in high school and college. Not only that but the girls on the sidelines looked like Bailey, Quinn, and Molly — my first middle school crushes. The assistant producers must have talked to my mom. She must have sent them pictures, and we must have one hell of a casting agency.

A helicopter hovered over the field, and I waited to see if it was going to land on the center circle. It didn't touch down straightaway, but that didn't mean it wasn't coming for me. Maybe they needed to take some aerial shots first, or maybe they were waiting for me to signal when I was done, or maybe it was just a preview of what was to come later. I was giddy thinking about who was in the helicopter with The Producer—Jay Z? Jermaine Dupri? Missy Elliott? Dave Chappelle? Jimmy Fallon? He knew all of them, and he'd promised to introduce me when the time was right.

I figured I'd better keep moving—we didn't need three hours of footage at the soccer field. I quickly spotted my next mark: a group of black guys standing in a circle on the corner and shooting the shit. A rap battle felt appropriate, so I came in and started spitting. My words spilled out of me as if I was reciting memorized verses, as familiar as the Pledge of Allegiance but faster and fiercer than Eminem. "Hot like the kettle when the pedal hit the metal, Pinocchio you know son of Geppetto, hello!"

It was straight out of a nineties music video, the whole squad dressed in Timberlands, baggy hoodies, and puffy coats; one of them even sucked on a dry blunt stick à la Method Man. "Yo, man. You gotta chill. You're gonna get squashed." I wasn't sure if he meant by him or the traffic.

"Nothing can touch me. This is my day," I said and threw my fitted Yankees cap on the ground—a demonstration of victory and a generous offering, since it would soon be a valuable souvenir. Everyone has a Bill Murray story. If that guy was smart and kept my hat, he'd have proof that he'd once battled Myles McDermott (my stage name).

"You're crazy, dude. You should roll. Be careful."

I sprinted back across Houston, to show the hip-hop crew that the city really was shut down for me. The drivers once again swerved to avoid me and each other while honking and yelling a realistic variety of obscenities. I considered popping into Katz's, the iconic deli where Meg Ryan and Billy Crystal shot their famous scene in *When Harry Met Sally,* but it seemed too obvious.

I ran through the city for the next ten hours, following my marks. At some point it occurred to me that eight million people lived in New York; even if we had Scorsese's budget, we couldn't afford to shut down the entire city. There had to be some real people mingling in and out of our production. But how was I supposed to keep the thread if no one told me what to do or gave me any direction?

I didn't have much time to think on it because the late, great "Macho Man" Randy Savage was leading a gang of bikers north on First Avenue. It's a straight shot to Yankee Stadium, that's why. And where was I three nights ago? Yankee Stadium. What happened when I walked in in the middle of the second inning? Jay Z, The Producer's crown jewel connection, was on the jumbotron. And what was the song they played when he popped up on-screen? "Brooklyn We Go Hard." So where to go? Brooklyn. And go hard.

But hold up. What if I was supposed to follow the bikers to Yankee Stadium? They didn't really expect me to walk to the Bronx, did they? I sat on the sidewalk and paused to think it over. I saw an upscale salon — that'd be the perfect way to touch up hair and makeup without halting the shooting. The motherfucking Producer thought of everything.

I walked into the salon and asked, "How much for a touch-up?"

"What's a touch-up?"

"You know…" I winked at her and made exaggerated air quotes. "Just the 'usual,' whatever that is."

She looked confused and said, "Well, trims start at two hundred."

Fuck that. Or maybe not — maybe The Producer was telling me that I would soon be able to afford $200 touch-ups. Or maybe he was giving a cost-prohibitive number. The character Myles McDermott couldn't afford a $200 touch-up; he's a public defender and a struggling comic, after all. I figured it meant I should get the fuck out of there and back on the streets—we don't need no damn haircut. Then the phone rang. She stayed on for way too long—*Time is money, woman*—and then told me, "I'm sorry, sir, but we just booked our final slot for tonight. Would you like me to make an appointment for you tomorrow?" Genius. Genius. Genius.

"Yes, indeed. Tomorrow it is, madam."

I walked out of the salon and made an important realization: The Bowery Hotel was two blocks away. I'd been in there a few weeks prior and seen either Mary-Kate or Ashley Olsen—don't know which one, doesn't matter. The Producer had built in a break for me because of course I'd be tired by hour nine. I could go take a load off, get a drink, even. Plus, that's where deals get made, and maybe I was there to make a deal.

I walked through the lobby—the only guy in soccer shorts, swag on another level. I didn't wait to be seated; I just walked past all the suits and socialites to the back patio. A waitress came over and asked me if I needed anything. "I was thinking about having a little champagne," I said, assuming she'd probably bring me a bottle of their finest. The execs around me spoke into their BlackBerrys in hushed tones. *He's here, what do you want me to do?* Maybe they were just checking out the goods today—the endorsement negotiations would happen on a future date. I didn't feel like talking business anyway, so I just started barking toward the microphones in the trees. "Just my mom. My mom and The Producer, if you want to come out. Those are the only people I want to see—no business right now. Art before money." The waitress was taking too long and I was losing steam, so I bailed.

I resumed following the flow of foot traffic through the East Village, still certain that the producers watching on monitors were using the pedestrians to guide me, still trying to solve the enigma of where the producers had set up their remote control room. *Where is the camera? iPhones can't be capturing all of this.* I ended up on a Brooklyn-bound L train headed to Williamsburg. I peeled off my shirt, grabbed the overhead bar, and started doing pull-ups on the train. We could use that for promos or B roll.

When the train stopped, everyone spilled out in their own directions. Half went left, half went right, and I didn't know who to follow. *How do I know where to go? How do I know when this is over?* I couldn't spot the eye in the sky. This was starting to feel less like a TV show and more like surveillance — a sick social experiment to see how far I'd go for the cameras. Alone and without guidance, I panicked. My eyes filled with tears. "What do you want from me?!" I screamed, crying so hard my contacts flushed out of my eyes. I'd lost the game.

Two NYPD officers approached. Their uniforms looked real. My hands were folded behind my head like a captured soldier. I was barefoot and shirtless, wearing only soccer shorts in late October.

"What's the matter, buddy?" the first cop asked.

"I don't know. I'm trying to figure it out."

"You're standing on a subway platform with no shoes on, no shirt, and you're crying. That don't seem like a problem to you?" The second cop seemed to be playing the role of Bad Cop.

"I think the problem is I'm cold."

"You don't seem violent."

"I'm completely nonviolent."

"So you don't mind if we just cuff you for safety purposes, then?"

"But you're not real cops?" I asked as they detained me.

"No, there's a costume party later."

Like the construction workers, their accents were just a little too authentic, and their radios were a bit overactive. They weren't real; I didn't need to invoke my Sixth Amendment right to counsel.

They led me to a tiny satellite office inside the subway station. "I don't suppose you have ID?" Good Cop asked.

"Not in my pocketless shorts, no."

I found myself in the back of an ambulance instead of a squad car. The paramedics told me we had to wait but otherwise seemed entirely uninterested in anything I had to say. They listened on the radio to the Yankees playing the Angels for the American League Championship, but it sounded prerecorded. And who under the age of seventy actually listened to baseball games? We were in a holding pattern, but for what I didn't know.

After three or so innings, another radio cracked on: "Intake available at Bellevue."

CHAPTER 2

NORMALLY I WASN'T THE guy riding in the ambulance to Bellevue. I was the guy who represented you after the police declared you an EDP — emotionally disturbed person — and decided that you need a visit to the psych ward before you're stable enough to go in front of a judge. Maybe you took a shit on the subway. Maybe it's the crack and the bugs are back. Maybe you were so high on meth you convinced yourself you were the devil and put two steak knives in your skull where your horns should be.

I was in my first year as a public defender in Brooklyn, and I'd already seen more than a hundred of these EDP cases. Earl Miller Jr. was the most memorable, and he wasn't just screaming at the wind when the police found him; Earl had a "landlord–tenant issue" on his hands.

Like all my clients, I first met Earl in "the pen" — one huge jail cell in the bowels of Brooklyn Criminal Court, reeking of homelessness, halitosis, piss, and moldy cheese sandwiches that no one eats. Night arraignments run until 1 a.m., and many in the pen — all black or brown, save an occasional drunk Russian — have been through the system enough times to know that if they don't get called before 1 a.m. they won't see a judge until the next morning. There's no rhyme or reason to the order in which they will see an attorney, and some have been sitting in the cage for twenty-four hours. Unsurprisingly, the possibility of a night upright on a cement bench doesn't result in a calm atmosphere: restlessness, desperation, and anger are as thick as the smell. Every name called pisses off the other twenty-nine men packed in like cattle.

"Earl Miller Jr."

An enormous man, probably thirty-six inches from shoulder to shoulder, squeezed into the interview booth. Before I could hand over my business card and say "Hi, I'm Zack McDermott. I'm going to be your lawyer," Earl was already shouting everyone's first question: "Am I going home?"

Earl Jr.'s head was shaved bald, shiny, and—like his shoulders—cartoonishly huge. His eyes were moist, large, and vacant; his cheeks so puffy it looked like he was holding his breath. But most people's attention would probably be drawn first to the scar that ran from his left eyebrow to just below his bottom lip. I couldn't imagine this man smiling. "Dis ain't nuttin but a landlord–tenant issue." His voice was deep and sluggish, like a bear that's been shot with a tranquilizer dart. I still hadn't given him my card; he was worked up enough that I decided to just skip it for the moment. "Landlord–tenant issue. That's all this is." The criminal complaint I was holding suggested otherwise.

"Earl, did you have a problem with your landlord?"

"That's all it fucking is."

"Okay. I understand you think this is a landlord–tenant issue, but you are in jail. Can I tell you what they are accusing you of?"

"You can't tell me shit because dis a landlord–tenant issue! You ain't my fucking landlord!"

"No, I'm your lawyer. And they—the cops and the DA—think it's more serious than that. The police are saying you threatened to burn down your apartment and that you had a bat or a club and you were threatening this guy, Daniel, saying you were going to fuck him up. Is any of that true? Did he threaten you?"

"I ain't talking to you."

"I think you should, because if you don't, I can't really help you, and no one else is trying to."

It was late in the night and if I was going to get Earl in front of the judge and possibly save him a night on Rikers, we were going to have to move.

"Five minutes, Counsel, the judge wants your notice!" a court officer hollered at me.

People who have been in and out of the system can usually detect bullshit pretty quickly, and normally I can get my clients, however belligerent they are at our introduction, to trust me. But I could tell Earl's distrust was different from the standard convict's contempt for every member of the system. He simply didn't know what the fuck was going on. I followed the script the PD's office taught us for cases like this.

"Earl, can you tell me if any of this stuff they are saying about you is true? I'm not saying it's true. It's the police's story. But can you tell me *your* story? We gotta move here. I have to ask you some questions, fast, if we're going to get you out of here tonight."

"Fuck you mean *if?!* Dis ain't nuttin but a landlord–tenant issue! I'm getting the fuck outta here! Just let me talk to the judge! Fuck outta here, man!"

He got up and slammed his meaty palm against the glass.

"Real quick, Earl: Have you ever taken any medication?"

"Yeah."

"Do you know what you take, Earl?"

"Seroquel."

"Anything else? Risperdal maybe? Depakote?" Knowing the names of the popular antipsychotic meds was part of the job—it came up a lot.

"Depakote."

"You ever been to the hospital for anything?"

"Yeah. I been to the hospital."

"Did they give you drugs there? Is that where you started the Depakote?"

"Yeah."

"Did they say maybe you were bipolar? Or schizophrenic?"

"Yeah. I been that."

"All right, thank you."

I scribbled "730?" on the top left corner of my file—shorthand for New York Criminal Procedure Law § 730.10, the statute that says any defendant who, as a result of mental disease or defect, lacks the capacity to understand the proceedings against him or assist in his own defense must have his case dismissed. That doesn't mean he gets to go home, though; best-case scenario, he'd end up at Bellevue psych ward instead of Rikers. Downside is, at Bellevue he'd still be among "criminals," and they'd *all* be mentally ill.

"One more thing. Don't talk to the judge. Don't say shit. Only I talk, okay? It's your only chance of getting out tonight."

"Fuck outta here, man."

"I'm serious. Nothing. If you have something you want to say, whisper it in my ear and I'll tell the judge."

Help us, patron saint of bail arguments, whoever you are. Shut Earl the fuck up for two minutes, in the name of all that is holy. Amen.

"Counsel, now or never." The court officer didn't appreciate me stretching the usual five-minute interview into seven.

Everything was fine in front of the judge…until Your Honor asked Counsel where, if released (and that's a big if), his client would be staying for the evening.

"He can stay with his mother, Judge."

"I need an address," the judge said.

I whispered in Earl's ear, "Give me an address. You can make it up. Just give me some numbers and a street. Make it your mom's if you can."

Armageddon. "Fuck outta here! Cocksucker! Tell this fucking

judge dis ain't nuttin but a landlord–tenant issue. I ain't gotta tell you no fucking address! This a illegal landlord!"

A fella Earl's size doesn't have to flail too long or too hard to get taken down by four or five court officers and dragged by his feet out of the courtroom and back into the pen. I took a little sidestep away from the lectern, just far enough to avoid getting gang-tackled along with him, but I kept a poker face in a feeble, nonverbal attempt to persuade the judge that *This ain't nothing to be scared of. Just a little ol' landlord–tenant issue.* In other words, *My dude's not a threat to society.*

"Judge, if I may be heard on bail."

"Counsel, just stop."

"But, Judge —"

Gavel.

"Enough! I'm done here. Bail is set in the amount of five thousand dollars."

Gavel.

"Judge, it's a misdemean —"

"AR-3 is adjourned for the evening and will resume at nine thirty tomorrow morning."

The crowd clucked and groaned. Their loved ones would be caged overnight.

"Counsel, a quick word?" The judge was all smiley now, off the record and on his way to a cab.

"Of course, Judge."

"Is he 730?"

"Off the record? Maybe."

Pretty switched on, that judge. Managed to deduce that something wasn't quite right with the flailing giant who could still be heard screaming "Fuck outta here!" from all the way back in the pen.

"I thought so, Counsel. Good night. Good job."

"Thank you, Judge. You too." *You indifferent cocksucker.*

*   *   *

I became a public defender to represent the dregs, the castoffs, the addicts, and the Uncle Eddies. People who come from the kind of poverty that makes them steal Tide from a Rite Aid to sell on the black market and puts them in the pen, in line right in front of Earl at night arraignments. My opponents: judges who take offense at profanity out of the mouths of schizophrenics; DAs who think the best solution for a guy like Earl—a man who could barely tie his shoes, let alone light a brick building on fire—is to lock him in a cage; cops who collar and drive the Earls of the world to Central Booking instead of the hospital.

I grew up in Wichita, Kansas, in a house that was a baloney sandwich throw from the trailer park. My mom, the Bird—a high school teacher with a passion for helping the "bad" kids—welcomed into our home any thug, gangbanger, ex-con, or other member of the general discard pile. When I was in high school, she tutored Crips and Bloods alike around our dinner table every day after school. Some got shot, some went to jail, some went to college. A couple did all three.

Watching my mom tutor eighteen-year-olds who read at a second-grade level—and who considered our humble abode the Taj Mahal because we had a weight bench and a Sega Genesis—showed me that the difference between the track to prison and the track to grad school boils down to roughly a thousand consecutive nights of *Clifford the Big Red Dog* and *Where the Wild Things Are,* along with being told by someone who loves you: "A writer is *always* writing" and "A writer's job is to tell the truth" and, once, "A writer is a liar. A *good* writer is a *good* liar. And you're a silver-tongued devil, boy." In other words, being lucky enough to have the Bird or someone like her as your mom.

Playing video games and pickup basketball in the driveway with guys who would graduate to federal prison introduced me to America's locking-black-men-in-cages phenomenon. I studied Malcolm X and Cornel West in college and started reading prison memoirs, which got me to thinking: *Isn't locking a man in a cage and subjecting him to beatings and possible rape and murder a tad harsh for selling a little dope?*

Law school was not only my ticket out of the lower middle class and out of Wichita, but also a chance for me to help keep the disadvantaged out of prison. I grew up on Natty Lights, mac 'n' cheese, and Camaro lust; I was never going to be a slick dick corporate lawyer drinking $17 cocktails after work and slamming my fist on the boardroom table. Researching contracts for the Koch brothers or Exxon held no appeal. No, my mission was to push back against the weight of racial injustice. Get my Malcolm X on.

While I never doubted that I'd picked the right hill to die on, even in my first nine months on the job, I couldn't help but wonder if I was too late to the battle. After crumbled communities, failed schools, narcotics, disease, prejudice, and disregard had done their work, I'd be lying if I said it didn't feel like I was trying to clean up the ocean one gum wrapper at a time.

Thankfully, the cure for soul-crushing impotence in the face of systemic injustice is laughter, and we public defenders are not above having a laugh at some pretty fucked-up shit. And in the modern penal state, once you get over the abject brutality, the brain-seizing injustice, and the rancid smell, there is plenty of comedy to go around. As a PD, even the average phone call is more colorful than the typical corporate lawyer's entire workweek.

"Hello. Legal Aid."

"This is Anne."

"Anne who?"

"Anne with the prostitution case."

"Anne with the prostitution case…"

"The one that they say I gave a blowjob for ten dollars behind the train station."

"Which train station?"

"Canarsie L."

Oh, $10-L-Train-Blowjob Anne. "Right, how are you? So sorry. Let me get your file. Hey, can you hold on really quick? Other line... Hello?"

"This Keith."

"Keith who?"

"Keith I had a case."

Right, Keith, figured. That's why you're calling me. "Which case?"

"They say I beat up my girlfriend and I got an order of protection now."

Right, Keith. I have twelve of those...

"It was my child's mother."

I have ten of those. "Any weapons involved? When did you get arraigned? When's your next court date? Can you give me your last name?"

Friends, strangers too, love to ask, "What's the most interesting case you have right now?" *I don't know.* "What's the most fucked-up?" *I don't know.* But then, when I think about my day for a minute, I realize that I can say with a straight face, "Yesterday a woman told me that of course she didn't have any crack rock. If she had crack rock, she'd have just put it in her pussy. "Why wouldn't I just put it in my pussy? Answer me that—if I had a rock, why wouldn't I just put it in my pussy?" It's a good question. Not sure I'd lead with it in front of the judge, but a valid point nonetheless.

So that was my nine-to-five: crack in the pussy, homeless people yelling at me, me begging DAs for plea bargains, me selling those plea bargains to the homeless people, piss-smelling jail cells, seizures at the lectern, power-tripping judges, and court officers yelling at mothers worried about their babies being sent to Rikers Island. I had a front-row seat to a fascinating and horrible postmodern moral-ity play starring drug addicts, cops, wannabe cops, crusading DAs, hippie antiestablishment anarchist colleagues, jaded and worn-down alcoholic colleagues, and a basketful of various other cautionary tales. I wasn't sure yet what my role in this production would be, but, Lord, it was horrendous, engrossing, and—if you looked at it right—mordantly entertaining.

I'd passed exactly five and a half hours in Manhattan before moving there, and three of those were spent interviewing for my job at Le-gal Aid. Everything I knew about the city came from TV, movies, and late-nineties hip-hop. *Seinfeld* taught me that I might be able to date out of my league; *Home Alone 2* showed me that the Plaza was a fine place to lay one's head; and Biggie and Jay Z informed me that, for a young and hungry public defender, Brooklyn was where the action was.

I lived in a half-dozen apartments with fifteen different roommates in my first year in New York. Every time I moved into a new place, I brought fewer and fewer possessions with me. By the time I settled into my apartment on St. Marks, I could fit everything I owned, along with myself, in a yellow cab; eventually it took just two hours to go from first T-shirt packed to housewarming party. It was exactly as glamorous as it sounds—both the good and the bad—but I was drinking New York from a fire hose.

First stop was Harlem with the Regis brothers. They had the same dad but different moms. Sian-Pierre was working at BET and starting a fashion blog. Joe was an investment banker. We smoked and watched *Planet Earth* after work every night with the girls next door. They became my first close friends in New York, but Harlem turned out to be too damn far from Brooklyn, even when I still looked for-ward to riding the subway every morning.

Next, I moved in with three young attorneys from my office who were a man short of signing a lease on a four-bedroom. That also lasted a month. I called it quits after one of them tried to fight me for declining his invitation to go shot for shot to the bottom of his half-empty liter of vodka; it was a Wednesday. I never complained that he and the other two blacked out four nights a week and occasionally smashed pint glasses against the wall. I didn't even mind their rampant cocaine use or their dealer buzzing himself up at 1 a.m. on a school night. But haze drinking at twenty-five was a bridge too far.

I found a little slice of serenity in Fort Greene with one gay male and one straight male. It took me two weeks to realize that Jon was actually the gay one. The reveal came when Jon saw me walking to the bathroom one morning in some fairly tiny boxer briefs and said, "You sure can wear a pair of underwear." Jon and Greg were fantastic, and they had a Roomba, but my room was way too small and I wanted to be back in the city, so that one lasted only two months.

My first East Village apartment followed, with a hard-partying fashion photographer roommate. The first Saturday I lived with him I came home at 4 a.m. to find him standing next to a pile of coke on our coffee table surrounded by a shirtless Frenchman and two girls screaming along to Queen's "Under Pressure."

Then it was a fifth-floor walk-up on the border of Chinatown and the Lower East Side. It was July, piping hot outside, and the unit had no AC. Most of our neighbors were Chinese, and much fish was cooked in underwear with open doors; eight or nine people in two-bedroom apartments. But I could live with the heat because my roommate was a gorgeous German girl with an amazing body who regularly walked around in her underwear. There was a *Streetcar Named Desire* level of sexual tension until we started sleeping with each other toward the end of the first week. That was also a one-month sublease, but we caught feelings, and before either of us knew it, we were reluctantly involved in a semi-monogamous relationship.

Union Square followed—there I lived with a French United

Nations intern. He idolized—and looked like—Henry Kissinger. I introduced him to marijuana and trap music; he became quite the fan of Three 6 Mafia. Our other roommate was tatted and ate prepackaged Trader Joe's sandwiches for almost every meal and blew through a couple of bottles of Two Buck Chuck every night.

In September I found what I thought would become a more long-term solution: a three-bedroom walk-up on the corner of St. Marks Place and Avenue A, above a not-quite-dive bar manned by an aspiring-actor-level good-looking Irishman. My roommate, Lucas, was the younger brother of my closest friend at Legal Aid. It sounds a little dramatic to label him a drug dealer—it was only pot—but that is how he paid his rent. So I guess Lucas was a drug dealer.

Most people living in New York on a limited budget end up migrating to Queens or Jersey. But while my vagabond lifestyle was partially a result of financial necessity—making it in New York on $50,000 a year requires some ingenuity—the real appeal for me was exposing myself to so many different people and lifestyles. Nearly everyone I met seemed to have a side hustle or dream job they were chasing, and hardly any of them exhibited even a hint of self-mockery about it. I quit smirking when I met waiters or bartenders who told me they were aspiring actors or musicians. It meant something different here; long-shot goals weren't the joke I historically took them to be. Members of iconic bands *did* start out bartending on the Lower East Side; future Hollywood stars *did* wait tables while they attended the Actors Studio. And, unlike in Wichita, no one here called you "queer" for pursuing a pipe dream.

In my case, the pursuit was stand-up comedy. Growing up, I had always preferred hearing "You're funny. Ever consider trying comedy?" to "You're an asshole that loves to argue. Ever consider becoming a lawyer?" But there's an easy-to-follow recipe for becoming an attorney: decent grades and LSAT score, $160,000 in law school loans, and scoring in the top seventieth percentile on the bar exam. The path to becoming a successful stand-up comic was a little harder to wrap my head around. But one month into living in New York I realized that I'd already inadvertently completed step one: move to New York. Step two: if you won't give it five years, don't give it five minutes. I had five years. Step three: get up onstage, every single night.

At first I approached stand-up like every other inexperienced comedian before me: stand on feet, ignore shaking hands and trembling legs, and nervously recite poorly crafted jokes scratched out the night before, striving for verbatim delivery. But then I realized, if I wanted to be good, I had to let my balls drop—be "me" onstage. Or, more accurately, I had to isolate and embody the craziest corner of my personality up there. And to do that I decided to method-act my way into that exaggeratedly crazy version of myself.

Thus, Myles McD was born. I couldn't use Zack as my stage name because I didn't want DAs to Google me and see me telling jokes about walking in on my mom riding her boyfriend Terry's BBD: "Get it, Terry, get it!" But professional reasons aside, while Zack might have had the potential to be a decent comic, Myles was an ace up the sleeve—a long-shot chance at making it.

Myles was the keyed-up, zero-shits-given version of myself. He was a sunglasses-at-night, no-underwear-wearing sort of prick. He had a Mohawk. He wore a handlebar moustache unapologetically. He didn't wear Zack's casual uniform of black T-shirts and sensible dark jeans with tennis shoes; he wore skintight retro tees, cutoffs, bandanas, and aviators.

As Myles, I spent the entire summer smoking pot and getting up onstage. On a typical night, I'd go to four or five open mics before starting the *real* work in front of the TV at one or two in the morning: joint and notepad in hand, watching first a documentary to mine material, then a stand-up special to study the pros. I was so locked in, sleep was a luxury I couldn't afford and didn't have time for.

I started calling clubs, "posing" as Myles's manager: "Can Myles come in and do a set tonight? He's working on a special and wants to tune up in some smaller venues."

"Who?"

"You ain't heard?!"

Unbelievably, it occasionally worked and I was able to steal some undeserved stage time as Myles. I still needed a game changer, though, if I was going to make the leap from up-and-comer to headliner.

I met The Producer early on in the open-mic circuit and we became fast friends. It was my second month in New York. I didn't know who he was at first, but it was clear he was *someone*. He didn't appear to have a regular job, but he lived in a swanky doorman building on the Upper West Side and dressed like a pop star. I had his rent pegged at five or six grand, his sneakers at the average retail price of $500 per, his leather jackets at probably close to a month's rent. He dressed like he had a stylist—newsboy caps and leather pants on occasion—and he seemed to never wear any of it twice. I knew he wasn't famous because I didn't even recognize his last name, but the outfits, the apartment, and the whole no-job thing lent him an air of celebrity.

We started hanging out at the Comedy Cellar together, and not just as patrons. For some reason, then unknown to me, we were allowed to sit at the legendary back table. The Cellar is a comedy mecca and the table is reserved exclusively for performing comics; it's not unusual for Chris Rock or Louis C.K. to post up. Basically, a seat there means you've made it as a comic. Within six months I'd gone from performing at crowdless open mics to rubbing elbows with the legends. Neither I nor Myles was close to being able to get onstage there yet, but it didn't seem outrageous to think the proximity signified something.

As it turned out, The Producer's sister was the famous one—a pop star who'd also been in some major films. I learned this information before he wanted me to—at a McDonald's, when he was recognized by the cashier.

The Producer had started out doing stand-up too, but eventually he phased himself out of performing and turned his focus and attention toward managing Myles. He'd introduce me to industry people as "the hottest up-and-coming comedian" and "my project" and "future star, Myles McDermott."

And there was some concrete proof that he meant it. After I finished the first draft of the pilot we were writing together, he rented out a space in Midtown where we held a casting call. Beautiful actresses lined up on folding chairs in the hallway, waiting to audition for the role of my girlfriend. They'd come into the room, read with me, and we'd say, "Okay, thanks. That was great." Everything was taped. It looked legit.

It all felt like I was being recruited. "As soon as I push the button, it's on. This will go fast. Be ready. I'm calling all my connects." I was practically frothing at the mouth for this button push, but my eagerness and single-minded focus came at a price. Initially, I had no problem switching back and forth between Zack and Myles, but as the months wore on, I became more and more consumed by my creation. Zack was dissolving.

Becoming Myles took a toll on my job performance. My intern that summer, Scott—a blue-eyed, baby-faced Minnesotan—might have known something was up. Normal duties for an intern include researching and writing motions, shadowing attorneys in court, and looking up homeless outreach programs and mental health services. I gave Scott two assignments all summer: (1) check my backlog of voicemails and transcribe my messages; and (2) accompany me to Best Buy and show me what HDMI cable I need to stream YouTube videos from my laptop to my TV while I smoke a joint and write jokes.

Assignment (2) was executed at 3 p.m. on a weekday, only minutes after he'd finished assignment (1). There were forty voicemails — about three full days' worth — but that's only because my mailbox was full. The messages were weeks old — DAs calling me to discuss plea deals, clients wondering why the fuck I hadn't called them back, defense attorneys from other offices looking to conference cases with codefendants. He scrawled them all out on a legal pad. I looked at the five pages of notes and said, "Fuck it. Let's go get that cable."

Before we got on the train to hit Best Buy, I told him we had to make a pit stop at Lids, the hat store. I wanted to get GUCCI inscribed on my fitted Yankees cap. The employee at the hat shop told me they couldn't do it. "It's trademarked." I argued with her, telling her it wasn't the brand I wanted but rather the name. Like the rapper Gucci Mane. What if my name was Gucci McDermott? She asked me if my name was Gucci and if I had any ID. I asked her if she knew anything about IP law. I told her Gucci Mane's name isn't really Gucci either. She said she wouldn't make it for Gucci Mane either. We went in circles for ten minutes, me growing increasingly livid and disrespectful.

When we left, Scott asked me, "Just how bipolar are you?" I took it as a compliment — the insinuation was a nod to my craftiness, as far as I was concerned. We got the HDMI cable from Best Buy and made our way to my apartment.

"I'm assuming *you* are the one who covered the walls in red Sharpie?"

"Scottie, hook up the HDMI cable and buckle up, would you?"

Then I showed a home video of me creating the masterpiece in question. I had been up until 4 a.m. the night before — using the white walls as my canvas and Nas as the soundtrack. I alternated between dancing half naked wearing a sombrero, writing jokes and poems on the wall, and crying. There was some spoken-word poetry as well.

I released Scott around 6 p.m. and thanked him for putting in such a long and productive day. "You have a trial tomorrow, yeah?" he asked on the way out the door.

"Ah, fuck. Yeah, man. Meet me at the office at eight forty-five? I'll prep you."

"Uh, okay. What's it about?"

"Ahhh, menacing with a knife. Old guy. Landlord. Not the crazy one."

Scott beat me to the office by a good half hour. "Scottie, let's boogie! Lionel Brown's freedom awaits." On the way to the courthouse, I handed him a legal pad and said, "Here, write shit down." Here's what Scott knew about the case: The older Jamaican fella, dressed in his Sunday best and seated next to us at counsel table, was our client; the fella was, maybe, charged with menacing; and Scott was supposed to write shit down.

What I knew was that the client was Lionel Brown, a seventy-something-year-old Jamaican man who had been coming back to court for almost a year because he refused to take a disorderly conduct plea. I knew he came to court dressed in his Sunday best every time. I knew he looked fantastic in his Sunday best. I knew I loved listening to his deep voice and slight Jamaican lilt. What I didn't know was jack shit about his case.

Judge Pickett drank a giant Arizona iced tea through a straw throughout the course of the three-hour bench trial. Lionel Brown laughed at the DA's questions. I cross-examined the landlord and got him to admit he wasn't afraid of LB when LB allegedly pulled the knife on him. "I ain't afraid o' nobody, man."

Not guilty.

We celebrated our victory at Legal Aid happy hour, which coincided with an LGBTQ recruiting event hosted by a white-shoe law firm. Since they had rented the place out and we were just crashing the party, the bartender told me we'd need permission from the firm to play any music. So I asked them. Request denied. Skewing 95/5 on the Myles/Zack meter, I put in my earbuds and cranked some Lady Gaga on max volume. "Scott, tape this." I unbuttoned my shirt halfway down my chest, slithered on my belly like a snake to the middle of the impromptu dance floor, popped up in front of a few of the sprightly young recruits, and started giving lap dances. Shirt came off; pants came off. There was some whooping from the crowd. There was some "This is not part of the event! This is not part of the show!" from the law firm stooges. The manager of the bar said she was going to call the police, which prompted me to give her a signature Chippendales gyration, pants still around my ankles. A fellow first-year attorney walked me out the door not long thereafter. No matter. I'd just received the text that would change my life for good.

Dude, how quick can you get to the Bowery Hotel?

Hour.

Come. Look like Myles. Meeting someone important.

I made it to the Bowery Hotel just before the arrival of whomever it was we were meeting. The Producer was outside chain-smoking Marlboro Lights. We hugged and I told him to give me a cigarette.

"This dude we are meeting with is the shit."

"Okay, who is he?"

"Just let me talk. You just sit there and be Myles. Don't say shit. Be funny."

"I can do that. But who the fuck is this?"

"He's a guy who's done a ton of shit. Just let me talk."

"I will. Give me another cigarette."

We smoked one more and grabbed a booth in the back. I kept my sunglasses on, like a dick. Our waitress dropped off menus and waters as our guest arrived. "Let me order," The Producer muttered under his breath right before our guy sat down.

"Eric, this is Myles. Myles, this is Eric."

We shook hands and I took my sunglasses off. Even Myles couldn't keep up that front for too long. "This is what I'm talking about," The Producer said, nodding in my direction.

"Okay, I can see it," Eric said.

"What are we seeing, gentlemen?" Both laughed too hard.

"That's him, man. That's it. That's Myles. You see what I'm saying?"

"Oh, I see it." Eric even sounded genuine somehow.

The waitress came over and The Producer ordered half the menu for the table.

"So Myles knows what you do. He knows your reputation. We want to pitch you some crazy shit. Basically, cross-country road trip, starring him obviously. Kind of a white-trash Ali G thing. This guy is like the young Larry David, but he's also from Kansas and he knows that world. We want to take him through the South, through the Midwest, and fuck with people. No script. He'll do whatever. He'll get arrested if that's what we need."

"I will. I'll do anything."

Eric nodded enthusiastically at everything The Producer said. My friend was the appeal, not me, not the idea. Still, I couldn't see beyond The Producer's enthusiasm. I thought I'd arrived.

Three days later, I walked out the front door of my apartment and into the pilot I knew we were shooting.

CHAPTER 3

IT SEEMED WEIRD THAT the paramedics followed me inside and stayed with me until I was escorted to an internal waiting room. Weirder still, every door I encountered was locked and required a series of maneuvers by a staff member to open.

A couple of homeless-looking guys nodded off in their chairs. There was a middle-aged white guy, built like my biological father: potbellied, slightly fatter, and with grayer hair. He had to have been cast to play Mack McDermott. My dad left when I was five and I hadn't seen him in a few years. The last time we parted ways, his right fist was cocked in front of my face as he slurred, "I should knock you the fuck out!"

The actor playing Mack looked sad, near tears. I patted him on the head, trying to console him. "Don't fucking touch me!" he yelled. I backed off but told him, "I'm here if you want to talk about it."

Simultaneously exhausted and restless, I paced the intake room, guessing at the purpose of this specific scene. *Are we even still shooting, or can the producers tell that I really need to see a doctor?* I was freezing. Maybe they were worried I'd get hypothermia. The medical equipment looked too expensive to break, so I decided against trashing it Mötley Crüe style. A green horizontal stripe, about the width of a man's size 11 shoe, was painted at waist height along the walls. I ran my hand along the stripe as I walked the corridor. *Green means go.*

"Bailey Wilmer, Klaus, Kewley and Keenan, my brother, my sister, the Jacobsons." I started listing people I was going to take care of once I made my fortune—friends from elementary school, the girl I'd lost my virginity to at fourteen, high school friends, people I barely remembered.

The purpose was twofold: (1) The Producer had promised me we were going to be rich beyond belief once we got our show off the ground. They needed a reminder that I was to be paid, and handsomely, for the shift I'd just put in—twelve hours, alone, in the cold, half naked, confused, searching for signposts, and now crying again. (2) Everyone needed to know just how brilliant I was. What a photographic memory I had. I rattled off at least fifty names inside of a minute, failing to repeat a single one or pause in the middle of a sentence.

Seinfeld was on TV. A fat white man stared at the screen, howling with laughter but clearly too drunk to understand the jokes. "Mack" sat next to him but kept his head down. He looked ashamed, probably reflecting on the missed birthdays and soccer games.

"Zachary McDermott? The doctor will see you now."

I was excited to see if it would be a real doctor or Dr. Dre. Did The Producer know him too?

"Zack, or Zachary?" The physician's assistant ushered me into a tiny exam room and told me to take a seat on the table. No fewer than six white coats lined the walls, shoulder to shoulder.

"It's usually Myles now, but, yeah, Zack's cool too. I know why I'm here. You want me to just flow a bit?"

"These are medical students. Do you mind if they sit in?"

The question seemed rhetorical. "Not at all. I get it. It's exciting to see this unfold."

"See what unfold?" the doctor asked.

"I realize now what those gifted tests in second grade were for. I intentionally gave wrong answers when they were testing me so they

34

wouldn't transfer me out of my big sister's school. But the tester knew, and he'd never seen a second grader capable of intentionally foiling the results. They told my mom my IQ was immeasurable."

"Lie down." The doctor's tone had shifted. He no longer seemed interested in analyzing the speed at which human neurons could fire inside the brains of the ninety-ninth percentile.

The medical students had filed out. In their place, three large black men encroached and circled me; their shadows congregated on my torso. A needle emerged, and the men crept closer.

"No needles! No needles! My uncle was a heroin addict! I can't do needles!"

"Just one," the doctor flatly answered.

The apparatus they used to pierce my arm looked nothing like any syringe I'd seen. It appeared to come from the future, shaped like a tiny *Star Trek* phaser, and it made the sound of a tire rapidly deflating as they injected me with something. Before I could decide if it was a tracking device or a computer chip, I was out.

I woke up on a different floor, wearing green scrubs. The patients from the intake were no longer there. A new cast of characters, also wearing scrubs, had replaced them. It seemed half of them had been told to pace the narrow corridor with just enough energy to remain upright, and the others to yell or sleep. A few did both at the same time. Many of these people appeared to be truly crazy. They certainly weren't breaking character. *Is it possible that we've secured permission to shoot in an actual psych ward?* I joined the walkers, but it was no more a conscious decision than a shark deciding to swim. The hall was narrow, claustrophobically so. There was no comfortable common room to take a load off. No decent furniture to sit on. Options were limited to pacing or lying in bed. I searched for clues as to whom, if anyone, I could trust to let me in on the game plan.

"You're Zachary M., right?" An orderly popped me out of my trance. "There's someone here for you."

Standing in the hospital's security vestibule, I spotted a middle-aged woman who looked a great deal like my mother undergoing an intense search and pat down. Her head pivoted from left to center to right, then back.

"Bird?"

I nicknamed her "the Bird" as a teen because of her tendency to move her head in these choppy semicircles when her feathers were ruffled. I squinted at her, trying without my contacts to make out the blurry image. Five foot one, large bosom, the exact same bushy eyebrows and bird beak of a nose as me. It checked out.

"Bird?" I asked as I approached. I wasn't certain it was her.

"The Bird is here," she said, looking me over.

"The Bird can't be here; the Bird lives in Wichita." I looked her over as well. The Payless shoes checked out. So did her hair color: black with highlights somewhere between purple and burnt red. She was put together, but her outfit probably didn't cost $50 head to toe. All signs pointed to this woman being the Bird, but she was shakier than usual. Trembling a little, even.

"The Bird got on a plane," she said. "You're a bag of bones, Gorilla."

It was when she used my nickname, born of my barrel chest and excessive body hair, that I fully accepted this was my mother and not an actor in prosthetics. Plus, if she were an actor, how would she know I'd lost thirty-five pounds in two months? I tried to step forward to hug her, but the orderly shouted, "Get behind the yellow line!" A decal on the ward's entrance read DANGER OF PATIENT ELOPEMENT. Nylon restraints peeked out of a supply drawer at the entrance.

We were escorted down the hall to the cafeteria at the back end of the ward, which doubled as the visitors' room. Mother and son required three orderlies and security personnel to supervise their conversation. One sat feet away on a metal folding chair, listening to every word we spoke.

"How'd you know where to find me, Bird?"

"The police told me."

"Police?"

"You gave them your brother's number. They called the house, said they'd found you on a subway platform and that you had no clothes on. All they would tell me was that they were taking you to a psych ward. Bellevue."

"I had shorts on. Where are you staying?"

"In your apartment. I saw the walls."

"What'd you think?" I felt like a renowned indie filmmaker, ready to field questions about the buzz surrounding his latest Sundance entry.

"You covered every inch of your walls in red marker, Zachary."

"I know." Why was this worrisome? Had she not seen the wall? It was brilliant:

A Fraction of the Whole =
Everything is Everything =
Wu-Tang =
36 Chambers + 5 =
41 Shots, We are all Amadou Diallo

The entire living room, kitchen, bathroom (mirror included), and my bedroom were covered in word equations.

"It reminded me of 'red rum, red rum,'" she said.

"I think you're thinking of *A Beautiful Mind*. Did you see the dad from *Everybody Loves Raymond*? He's here." I pointed to the old man shuffling down the hall just outside the cafeteria. My mom started to laugh but stopped abruptly when I didn't join in.

"He *looks* a lot like the old man from *Everybody Loves Raymond*, but that guy is just another patient here."

I huddled closer to her, deciding it was time to let her in on the secret. "There are no patients here. These people are actors. It actually *is* him." I was beaming.

"That guy died years ago."

Clearly the producers had decided not to tell her what was going on in order to keep her performance authentic.

"Mom, you're a terrible actor."

"Zack. You. Are. In. A. Locked. Psychiatric. Ward." She paused between each word.

"There are maybe *some* patients here, but most of these people are actors. Call my partner, my producer buddy. He'll explain what's going on." I pointed to a security camera mounted on the ceiling, which provided all the explanation needed, but I sensed she was still unpersuaded. "If I wasn't being filmed, then why was Daniel Day-Lewis on my block?"

"Son, I spent twenty minutes in your neighborhood, and half the people on your street look like Daniel Day-Lewis."

I stared at her.

"And I did call your producer buddy. He said you hadn't been sleeping for weeks and that he made you see a doctor before he'd continue working with you. I also called his mom. She hung up on me."

I kept staring.

"What about the Mohawk?" she asked after a silence. "Since when are you the Mohawk type?"

"Since my buddy shaved it. It's for comedy. For my act. For *this*. It's not funny to you?"

The Bird took my hand. This breed of bird does not shrink from adversity.

CHAPTER 4

BEFORE SHE WAS THE BIRD, she was Cin-Cin McGilvrey. The good kid and the peacemaker at home—she made deals with the Lord that if she colored perfectly between the lines of her Winnie-the-Pooh coloring books, her dad wouldn't get drunk. Her homework was done, and perfectly, without asking. By the time she started fifth grade, she'd burned through a great deal of the seventh-grade titles in the library. It didn't change things, though.

Every Friday Pa would leave to "get a gallon of milk and a loaf of bread." Granny would nod and exhale through her nostrils. Once Cin-Cin tried to call bullshit: "But the gallon in the refrigerator isn't even half empty yet!" Pa cleared his throat. Granny looked at Cin-Cin and then her husband—*Go ahead,* she seemed to say. *Since when do you need my permission?*

Cin-Cin didn't know where he went, only that when he came home he had transformed into a bear. And not a fun circus bear, an angry North American grizzly bear. Her bedroom was directly across the hall from her parents' room, and on Friday nights Granny would warn the family bookworm not to read under the covers and to go right to sleep. Cin-Cin wanted to leave her door open, curious as to what would happen when the bear returned, but Granny always shut it before she went to bed in her own room. Watching through her bedroom window, Cin-Cin would catch the bear sneaking in late.

She'd hear his keys jangling in the lock; sometimes it'd take him ten minutes to get the door open. He'd curse and stumble the entire time. "Goddamn door. Goddamn keys." He'd drop them, pick them up, drop them again. Curse some more. Now he really looked like a bear: awkward on his hind legs, not quite sure how to use them. It wasn't unusual for him to fall.

When my grandma heard him, she'd race to look out the back door to make sure the car made it into the driveway. Then she'd run back to her bedroom. Cin-Cin would peek her head out into the hallway. "Momma, what are you doing?" Granny would shout-whisper, "Get back in bed. Go back to sleep. Don't let your father know you're awake." Despite being fall-down drunk already, Pa would make a pit stop on his way to bed, crack another beer, and smoke another Salem. Cin-Cin knew she'd have seven minutes before the ugliness in the next room began. She pleaded with God for them to get divorced, or worse.

Pa would poke toward the bedroom, knocking knickknacks off the walls along the way. Granny would pretend to be asleep, but Pa would flick the bedroom light on anyway. Cin-Cin would hear him try to undress while he continued to stumble around. "Don't pretend like you're asleep," he'd tell Granny. "I'm sick of your holier-than-thou, high-horse attitude. *Your* dad and *your* farm and *your* kids." They were his kids too, but the world turned against him on Friday evenings.

"William, please, you're going to wake Cindy up."

"T'hell with Cindy," he'd say. "T'hell with Boeing. T'hell with you. I'm tired of being kicked around."

One particularly bad Friday night she heard Granny cry out, "Don't, William! Please! You're drunk!" followed by the sound of the big oaf collapsing onto the bed. Cin-Cin wandered into the hall, Winnie-the-Pooh in hand, and saw her father stumble from the bedroom. He looked like Humpty Dumpty in his boxer shorts. Her mom was sobbing in the other room as Pa hurled pots and pans against the wall in the kitchen. She knew it was almost over when she heard the cellophane crumple of his Salems and the click of his silver Zippo.

Soon he'd be en route to his corner chair, where he'd pop one last Miller Lite and smoke until he passed out. Granny must have also listened for the cellophane and the lighter flick, because she seemed to know exactly how long to wait before going to survey the mess Pa had left in her kitchen.

The North American grizzly remained ensconced in his cave for the greater part of that Saturday morning, snoring away. Cin-Cin crept into the kitchen, expecting maybe to find lingering evidence of the demolition she had pretended to sleep through. Instead, Granny was reading the newspaper and sipping coffee, the kitchen in perfect order. "Good morning, Cin-Cin. Shall I fix you cinnamon oatmeal or pancakes?"

Cin-Cin wanted to yell at her mom, tell her that she wasn't stupid or deaf, and to beg her to leave. Granny might have wanted to, but she'd no sooner divorce him than run away and join a cult. The best Cin-Cin could muster was "Daddy was scary last night." To which Granny replied, "Cinnamon oatmeal or pancakes? You are far too sensitive, Cin-Cin." She ordered pancakes, and while she waited for Granny to prepare her breakfast, she surveyed the freshly mopped linoleum floor. She noticed a brown indentation in front of the refrigerator—it looked like a smashed, twisted caterpillar. Sparkling floors were not low on Granny's list of priorities. "Mom, what happened?" She pointed at the caterpillar. Granny grimaced but explained, "It's nothing. Daddy just dropped his cigarette."

When Cin-Cin returned her focus to the new hole in the kitchen wall, Granny nudged her out of the house and gave her money for a Tastee-Freez. So Cin-Cin made her way to her friend Shellie's. Shellie's dad was up, and he was cooking breakfast in a goofy chef's hat while her mom lounged in her bathrobe. Shellie was embarrassed, but Cin-Cin wanted to trade.

The bear was up when she returned a few hours later. "Hi, Cindy-snoots," he greeted her as she walked in the door. Pa was showered and shaved and inevitably smoking. In the light of day, he was no longer a grizzly bear but a giant pink-eyed rat. "How'd you like to run errands with me today? We need to get your mama some flowers. How about you help me pick them out?" Despite his hangovers, he was nicest on Saturday mornings — sheepish and remorseful, although probably not certain for what.

My parents started dating when they were thirteen years old. The relationship got off to a rocky start. Valentine's Day, Mead Middle School, 1974: Mack was supposed to bring the Bird a "love ring" and ask her to go steady, but he didn't even make it to school. She was humiliated. On February 15, Mack did make it to school, ring in tow. He was stoned, his hair was greasy, his blackheads were in full bloom, and he smelled like BO. She gratefully accepted his ring and his apology. "I was sick and I missed the bus. I woke my mom up and asked her to take me to school, but she went back to sleep," he claimed. She bought the sick excuse — he was either exhibiting symptoms or doing a fine job of faking a sinus infection — but the mom sleeping part was beyond her comprehension. *Aren't moms supposed to be alarm clocks? To pack lunches, make beds, braid hair, help with homework, and lay out ironed outfits the night before school? This poor boy…His momma doesn't love him.* The Bird resolved to take care of him: she did his homework and gave him half of her lunch every day. Mack told her about his father, who ordered him to cut his hair and called him a worthless hippy. "You're lazy, lazy, lazy," my future grandad would say. "Lazy as a two-legged coon dog without a job."

Middle school relationships usually have a natural termination point — the young lovers go to different high schools or turn fifteen and realize they aren't soul mates after all. That's not how it shook out for my parents. They got married at eighteen. It would have been sooner but they decided to put off tying the knot until after they graduated high school. My mom graduated near the top of her class, and earned Mack a decent but semi-believable GPA.

Granny and Pa weren't pleased. Eighteen was young to get married, even in Kansas in 1978, and Mack was the sort of fella no one needed to catch in the act to know that he liked to party. Straight-A Cin-Cin was no rebel, but she was in love.

Six months later, and not at all on purpose, my mom was knocked up with Alexa, my older sister. The Bird had just finished her first semester of college and, even though she'd made the dean's list, didn't give much thought to her decision to drop out of school. The boy who'd been late with the love ring had not improved in the reliability department. Someone was going to have to raise the kid and support the family. She transferred to Dillon's grocery store.

By this time Mack was snorting coke something serious. Which, surprisingly, was not on the Bird's radar. She knew he could twist a joint one handed while driving, and she knew he could put down a few rum and Cokes, but cocaine was one of the few devils she didn't know. Pots and pans against the wall, shouting and perpetual grumpiness, yes. A brother high on PCP standing naked in the shower in front of his mother and attempting to eat a pickle jar, yes. But the occasional nosebleed didn't set off any alarm bells. At the height of his cocaine use, my dad was putting something like $800 a week up his nose. They were on food stamps.

Mack started asking strange favors from the Bird: he'd send her to FedEx with large cylindrical tubes meant to hold rolled-up photographs (oddly enough, he was a pretty good amateur photographer) and instructions to ship them to Florida. She didn't ask what was in the packages, but they sure were heavy for photos.

She could no longer deny that she was complicit in *something* once the house was burglarized by drug dealers. That night Mack came home at 3 a.m. to find the front door wide open, the living room window smashed in, his stereo and speakers gone, and his drum set knocked over. Alexa was running a high fever, and the Bird, nine months pregnant with me, was contemplating taking her to the hospital. Mack refused to call the cops and called her a "worrywart," as though she were stressing over who'd tracked mud all over her carpet.

Soon a new threat emerged and the worrywart started sleeping with a hammer on her nightstand. A few years before, the Bird had been forced to testify against Bert, one of Uncle Eddie's druggie friends (not that Uncle Eddie had any non-druggie friends), after he smashed in the front door of my parents' first apartment. He'd been running from the cops and wanted my mom to hide him. She refused, the landlord pressed charges for destruction of property, and the Bird was subpoenaed to testify.

Now, years after the trial, Bert was out of prison and harassing my mother. He'd leave her alone for months at a time, then he'd go on a drug binge and come looking for her. When she was pregnant with Adam, my little brother, Bert once pushed her against a sink in the back room of Dillon's bakery and told her, "I'm going to drag you into an alley and stick a knife in your belly." If Mack's truck wasn't in the driveway, Bert sometimes pounded on the front door hard enough to rattle the dead bolt: "I've been watching you! Let me see that baby! I'm going to get you!" The Bird would tell Mack, "The midnight caller paid us a visit again." "That's why you let the dog in at night," he'd remind her. My mom called the cops on Bert half a dozen times. Sometimes she couldn't help but fantasize that he would hurt her. That would serve Mack right — come home and find us all killed. But she stayed.

The house *itself* posed another danger. Mack was forever in the middle of a remodeling project. He never finished any of them. Our house was about as childproof as a steel mill. Tack strips lined the floors where he pulled up but did not replace the carpet. The "walls" were nothing but exposed insulation; Sheetrock leaned against the yellow fuzz but was never hung. Power saws, power sanders, nail guns, and paint cans were strewn about the floor. We had mice infestations so severe that the Bird frequently found nests. After she stepped on a mouse corpse and screamed, Mack told her to "quit being a baby." She laid poison throughout the house and launched a mouse genocide. After Granny told her not to leave poison out on the floor with toddlers running around, she subbed in mousetraps. So many mouse necks were snapped in that house that some days it sounded like the rodents honored their dead with twenty-one-gun salutes.

This was not how life was supposed to start for Cin-Cin.

Her parents, despite growing up dirt poor and shoeless in rural Oklahoma during the Great Depression, both graduated from Oklahoma A&M. Granny majored in being a secretary. Pa majored in business. My mom seemed a lock to keep the tradition going. Reading and writing had been her refuge from the liquored-up grizzly, straight A's through high school her offering to the gods to make it all stop. But it wasn't all just an escape—she genuinely loved literature and poetry. She dreamed of becoming an English teacher like Mrs. Ducroux, her favorite, who pulled books specifically for the Bird and who, when she caught the Bird reading a copy of *To Kill a Mockingbird* hidden in her third-grade textbook, told her she might want to secretly read something a little more age appropriate and led her to *Little House on the Prairie*. Every fall, when the college course catalogs were released—a reminder that she was missing yet another semester—the Bird's heart nearly exploded. In the end, she became the best-read grocery store doughnut fryer in Wichita.

Three kids and a man-child made reenrolling seem impossible. But even though Mack mocked her when she read and occasionally told her, "For someone who's supposed to be so book smart, you sure are stupid sometimes," he agreed to "babysit" if she wanted to take night classes. This lasted one semester. She had to pull out of half her courses because most nights he was late or high or both when his babysitting shift was supposed to start. She dropped out again.

She'd been all set to file for divorce in 1985. But then, broken rubber — third kid on the way. She was devastated. At the time, it was illegal in Kansas to get divorced while pregnant. Mack was happy. He was in one of his Jesus phases, taking the family to the Church of Christ — his dad's holy-rolling, dance-prohibiting, taking-the-Word-literallying, buffet-economy-stimulating Baptist church.

The Bird didn't go for the Baptists. Growing up, she'd spent her Sundays at Saint Margaret Mary. Even Pa rolled off the rack and made it to Mass on Sundays. Cin-Cin sat between her parents, a human buffer between Granny's stewing and Pa's boozy stench. She missed the weekly tradition, but Mack called Catholicism hocus-pocus. While she resented the elders at the Church of Christ imploring her to "be a more dutiful wife and take care of your husband's needs," Mack was nicer in his religious phases and a better father. It didn't curb his drug use at all, but it did make him think he wanted to save the family, and he solicited my five-year-old sister's help: When the Bird came home to find them playing horsey one evening, Alexa said, "Don't make my daddy leave. It's better when Daddy is here."

He had early warning of the Bird's intentions — he'd tapped the phone and recorded her calls for the better part of their final year together. The Bird figured it out after my dad forgot that one shouldn't use knowledge gained surreptitiously if one doesn't wish to be outed as a spy. He gave himself up with something like "And why are you so convinced I'm sleeping with Courtney?"

Finally, in 1988, she filed. Mack was ahead of her every step of the way — he still had the tape recorder hooked up in the basement. On his way out the door, my dad took $2,000 of the $2,037 in the checking account — money they'd set aside to buy new windows.

She and Mack had been married for ten years and together for half their lives. Even though she'd been thinking about leaving him on and off since before they were married, my mom wanted to kill herself. She wrote in her journal: *I felt like I had ruined Mack's life, taken my kids' daddy away, and cost my parents thousands of dollars. I was not only broke but in debt. My house was in shambles. I wanted to die. I didn't want to be a mother. But I didn't want Alexa to find my body. I didn't want to break my mom's heart. I thought and thought about suicide. I wondered who would raise my kids. I looked for Valium but didn't know if that was strong enough. I felt like the pain was never going to end and that I'd accomplished nothing. I couldn't find the pills.*

She was twenty-eight years old, with a two-year-old, a five-year-old, an eight-year-old, and $37.

CHAPTER 5

REGAINING SANITY IN A mental hospital is like treating a migraine at a rave. People screamed all day and night. The dad from *Everybody Loves Raymond* and I could barely lift our heads — he too sported a toddler's bib of drool on his shirt. A large African American woman — even the 4XL tops could not contain her — was always hysterical. For minutes at a time, she would wail at the top of her lungs, screaming, crying, spitting nonsense: "They're coming! They're coming for all of you! They gonna cut us open!" Even in Times Square, she would have attracted an audience. But in a psych ward, these types of hysterics are completely disorienting. Twenty souls lumped in together, dosed and ignored, all taking cues from one another. Each nonsensical tirade could alter the plot.

And it did. As we tried to piece together our own version of reality from a set of psychotic premises, paranoia came out of the woodwork. We speculated as to whether our food was being poisoned or whether the pills we were given were actually truth serums. Half of us did think we were pawns in some government plot, one step away from having our brains cut open.

My initial certainty that I was being videotaped was buoyed by the fact that the place looked exactly like the set of *One Flew Over the Cuckoo's Nest:* white walls, inmates wandering around drooling, belligerent patients tackled and injected. The only change since the

1950s seemed to be the smoking ban. There was one TV in the common room and arguments would break out — often escalating to the point of violence — over whether we should watch *Wendy Williams* or *Family Feud*. A black woman with an accent, possibly Haitian, once threatened to kill everyone in the room if *Wendy Williams* was changed one more time. She appeared capable. "I will lay hands on you motherfuckers!"

To avoid the mob, I continued swimming with the sharks — the group of patients whose daily activity consisted solely of pacing the corridor, end to end, for hours. A young African American patient — "Bone Crusher" he called himself — swung his fists back and forth and stomped down the hall, yelling "Bone Crusher! Bone Crusher! Bone Crusher!" Occasionally he'd take a break from the bone crushing to rap "Jesus Walks." Sometimes I stomped the halls and rapped along with Bone Crusher. Every time the N-word came around in the song, he tilted his head at me and I skipped a bar. In more sedated moments, I'd feel the top of my scrubs get wet and realize that a river of spit was coursing down my chin. Matching wet spots painted the crotch of my pants — the result of being too drugged to properly shake off.

At chow time, several five-foot-by-three-foot metal boxes were wheeled into the cafeteria, and chaos ensued. "Where the fuck is my food?!" about half the room would scream before the first tray was unloaded. The other half appeared completely unaware of our agenda in the cafeteria, oblivious to the fact that this would be our last opportunity to eat for hours.

In theory, each of us was to be fed according to our own specific dietary needs and restrictions. But there was no stopping the black market. Brazen hand-to-hands took place right out in the open.

"You gonna eat your roll? Hey, new motherfucker, I said you gonna eat your roll!"

"Yeah, I'm gonna eat my roll," I growled. I figured prison rules applied: cave once, bitch for life. But I wasn't opposed to a little horse-trading. "Can't do anything for you on the roll, but I will give you my cookie for your milk." A deal was struck, but it turned out I'd low-balled myself. Cookies were precious, and it was possible with a little begging to get an extra milk off one of the staff.

On my fourth day I learned there was something called Roof Group. *You mean to tell me we can go outside?* Technically, yes, but I learned that I personally could not go outside because I had to earn that privilege. Admittance to Roof Group—i.e., access to fresh air—required two weeks of good behavior and attendance at poorly advertised group therapy sessions.

And make no mistake about it: the air inside a psych ward is among the stalest and foulest on earth; 90 percent of our prescribed medications came with rancid and constant dog farts as a side effect. I needed that Roof Group, but goddamn—two weeks? Here?

So how to get out of this shit hole? Escape seemed impossible. The windows were strong, and we were at least twenty floors up. I knew I could slide out the first door where the visitors came in, but the two vestibule doors were never unlocked at the same time. Or I could get arrested.

I could get arrested. That's genius.

If they arrested me, they would have to take me to the precinct to process me. They would mark my commit card MEDICAL ATTEN-TION, meaning I wouldn't even have to wait in a cell for twenty-four hours. They'd bring me to arraignments, and I'd call Jonas Jacobson, my friend at work and probably the best trial lawyer in our office. He'd negotiate a favorable disposition and I'd be in and out before the night was over.

Okay, so what crime to commit? Assault in the Third Degree § 120.00(1) seemed easiest. Just hit someone. But who? Raymond's dad? Too old. Double Nightgown? Too crazy. Nurse? Too likely to cooperate with the prosecution. Can't do anything violent; that's stupid. Can't steal either; there's nothing to take.

Criminal Mischief in the Fourth Degree § 145.00. *A person is guilty of criminal mischief in the fourth degree when, having no right to do so nor any reasonable ground to believe that he or she has such right, he or she: (1) intentionally damages property of another person.* That should do it. Don't even need to go beyond sub (1). But what to damage? Everything is bolted down. The only pieces of furniture are plastic chairs. The TV is locked up and the pay phone is indestructible; plus, I'd probably be killed by the others if I fucked with either of those amenities. If I broke the window to the nurses' station, that would probably cause more than $1,500 in damage. That's a D felony. Shit, that's one to seven.

Six days in, I was still struggling to find a foothold in my new reality; I still hadn't quite found the game. Maybe the Bird was right: maybe this was psych ward qua psych ward. Maybe the reason she was a terrible actor was that neither she nor I was actually an actor. Maybe those security cams were closed-circuit. All I knew was I needed to get the fuck up out of there.

"How do I get the fuck up out of here?" I asked my favorite Haitian orderly.

"You have to ask to leave, and don't be nasty, man. You better than that."

Oh. Right. Of course I had to ask. I was being held *involuntarily*. A hospital doesn't have the right to kidnap you. No crime necessary.

"Give me a piece of paper."

I, Zachary McDermott, am demanding my release from this facility, Bellevue Hospital, on the 30th day of October, 2009. I affirm that I am not a danger to myself or others and that I am being held here against my will in violation of New York State law.

I felt pretty smug after ripping off that little missive. *Don't fuck with me. I'm a lawyer.* I also felt stupid because I'd relayed that standard many times to mentally unfit clients who'd been sent to jail *from* the psych ward: The hospital can place you on a seventy-two-hour hold if they believe you are a danger to yourself or others. They don't have to prove that you are at that point; they just have to say it. After that, you can request your release and you are entitled to a hearing, but the seventy-two-hour clock doesn't start until you make the request.

"You know I'm a lawyer?" I told the orderly, hoping he might pass that on to whoever mattered.

"I hear you saying that, but I don't know. You in here, man."

My demand for release was added to my file and, I imagined, docketed for discussion at the next staff meeting. But bureaucracy is slow, and no one was in any particular rush to get me out the door. There was still time to kill.

On day seven I walked by the activity room and noticed a fellow patient, a young Mexican guy, holding a pair of electric clippers and apparently giving out haircuts. He caught me staring.

"You want a haircut, man?"

"I guess?"

He sat me down and, without consulting me on what style I'd like, buzzed everything down to a two guard. No more Mohawk.

"You want me to hit your moustache too?"

"Sure."

He clipped the corners of my handlebar. The result left me looking less sinister, something approximating "normal," but I was still grasping for meaning. *Is this The Producer's plan? Does he want me to look more normal so we can further the plot and move the setting out of the psych ward?* If so, it would make sense to have another patient give me the cut — they could keep rolling and it would make for a funny, if head-scratching, scene. Why else would a patient in a psych ward be allowed to cut another person's hair?

On the other hand, maybe a Mexican guy cutting the hair of a fellow patient in a psych ward was just a Mexican guy cutting the hair of a fellow patient in a psych ward. Either way, I figured, it was good to hedge my bets. *If* there was a show and *if* the show wanted me out of this place, I was taking direction. *But* if I was really committed to a psych ward, I had to start working my way out. *And if this is all a game, why would the Bird be in New York this long? Why does she always look so upset, and why is she so insistent that this is real?*

I looked forward to the Bird's visits, but there were only two hours per day during which she was allowed. Every minute of every visiting opportunity, she was there. Ten minutes early, lined up at the door, ready to go through security — she was there. She didn't panic. Not in front of me. "What'd you have for lunch? Can you read anything? What are they making you do?" I couldn't really tell her; I was in a drug-induced fog, unable to distinguish one interaction from the next.

She wanted the staff to know I was not the man they saw. "This is not my son," she'd say. "*This* is my son," and she'd flash photos she'd brought with her of me looking "normal." To humanize me — to let them know not to discard *this* one. *He is loved. He's coming back. Help him.*

Just before my seventy-two hours ran out, I was called into a tiny office adjacent to the DANGER OF PATIENT ELOPEMENT doors. The Bird sat in on my discharge meeting. Her face said, *Don't screw this up. Don't be a smart-ass.* A young pretty doctor and an older nurse sat opposite us.

"Zachary, we understand you want to be released."

"I do."

"We aren't sure you're ready."

"I am. This place is hell."

"Your mom has agreed to take responsibility for you."

"Great."

"We need to discuss your diagnosis."

"I'm listening."

"You are bipolar and you had a psychotic break. You are currently on Depakote and Risperdal. Both will help you remain stable and avoid psychosis. It's imperative that you stay on these drugs. Do you understand that?"

"Question."

"Go ahead." Pretty Doctor was mildly annoyed.

"I can't feel my penis. I tried to masturbate the other day and I was completely numb. I can't feel anything, and I can't get hard."

"Do you want me to leave, Zack?" The Bird didn't really need to hear all this.

"No, cat's out of the bag."

"That's the Risperdal." Pretty Doctor could not have been more blasé. She wasn't the least bit concerned about the collateral damage to my penis.

"Okay, but...that doesn't really work for me."

"You might not need to take it forever."

"Okay, but...I might? So that doesn't work for me."

"Zack, you had a psychotic break. Honestly, if your mother wasn't willing to take full responsibility for you, there's no chance we'd be considering releasing you at this point. You don't seem to think this is a big deal, and we don't think you understand what's happened to you."

The Bird jumped in. "I am going to take him to Wichita as soon as he is released. He will be under my care, and he will be closely supervised. I have already lined up psychiatric care in Wichita, and I know that he will fully comply with his drug regimen. I will make him."

Reluctantly, Pretty Doctor handed over some paperwork. "You need to read and sign these forms. Again, I wouldn't even consider this if not for your mom and the after-care plan she's set up."

For the Bird, there was relief in the diagnosis. I *wasn't* schizo-phrenic like Uncle Eddie. There was hope that, if properly medicated, this could be an isolated incident. I furiously signed the stack of documents anywhere I could find a "signature_____ date_____."

"Okay, done."

"You didn't read anything." Pretty Doctor was now definitely an-noyed.

"I can speed-read. Do you want to test me for comprehension?" Warning sign: delusions of grandeur still present.

"Zack, don't be an ass." The Bird wanted me out of there, and quick. She seemed nervous that the whole thing could fall apart at any minute.

"Okay, I think we're good. Can my flaccid penis and I be on our way now?"

I'd forgotten what the sun felt like. It was better than I remembered, and I wanted to soak up as much as possible before it got dark outside. We decided to make the eighteen-block trip back to my apartment on foot.

That Manhattan is loud and fast is hardly news, but after a week with the zombies it felt like the Indy 500 was being raced on the street and the New York City Marathon was simultaneously under way on the sidewalk. Dizzying. I needed the Bird with me; there was no way I could've navigated it alone.

We walked the final few blocks back to my apartment, retracing in reverse the beginning steps of my TV shoot. Outside the little Aus-tralian meat pie spot on my corner, I suddenly remembered that, on my jaunt, I'd hoisted their five-gallon water jug over my head, fully intending to smash it through the window. I was saved only by the Aussie waitress, who gently said, "Don't, mate."

I looked across Tompkins Square Park and stared at the basketball court. *Could Daniel Day-Lewis really have been there? Could he really not have? Occam's razor says what?* I decided I didn't need to know right away.

The walls of my apartment were still covered in red Sharpie. Anyone — even I — could see that a tornado of madness had blown through here; the wreckage was everywhere. Twelve days earlier, I had been proud enough of my work that I'd expected my roommate to thank me when he saw it. I didn't understand when he sighed and went back to his room in a huff.

And, holy shit, it wasn't just my pothead roommate who'd seen all of this — I'd brought my fucking intern from Legal Aid into this place! Worse, I'd also shown him a good chunk of the ten hours of home video I shot while wearing a sombrero, first dancing and then crying. *What was Scottie thinking while he sat next to me at counsel table the next day?*

I paced my apartment for a few more minutes and went into the bathroom. I looked in the mirror and saw a stranger. My metabolism had been burning like a furnace for months from not sleeping or eating. I'd thought I looked ripped, but now it was clear I was just emaciated. The dark circles under my eyes were so pronounced it looked like I'd been punched. I'd aged five years in a few months.

My pupils were huge, dilated beyond belief. The pretty doctor's voice saying the words "psychotic break" played through my head on a loop. These eyes *looked* psychotic. Something was not right with the face I was staring at. *I had a psychotic break. I had a psychotic break. I had a psychotic break!* I was now in the same league as Charles Manson and Uncle Eddie. Eddie was the scarier proposition — we looked similar enough that it felt like he was staring back at me from the mirror. *Psychotic. You are psychotic.*

I wanted to shatter the glass. I wanted to bleed. But instead I collapsed in the corner. The incomprehensibility of the situation overwhelmed me. There was no TV show. I'd become a fucking crazy man.

The Bird came in and rubbed my back.

"I'm insane," I sobbed.

"You're going to be okay, Gorilla," she said.

"Psychotic!"

"You're okay."

"Have I been crazy my whole fucking life?"

"No, baby. You are okay. This is going to pass."

We flew home to Wichita the next morning.

CHAPTER 6

IN 1989, WHEN SIX-YEAR-OLD me watched the Bird walk into our small A-frame house—a $19,000 box with a triangle on top—after a long day at work, he saw a tired young woman in oversized round glasses, hair either in a perm or due for one, the straps of her brown Dillon's apron dangling at her sides. Her weariness was palpable to me even then.

The day the letter from Grow Your Own Teacher came, she tore it open while standing at the mailbox, then took off running down the block, yelling, "I got a scholarship! I got a scholarship!"

"What's a scholarship?" I asked. I'd never seen her that happy before.

"A scholarship means I am going back to school."

That sounded weird. "Will you wear a backpack?"

"I will wear a backpack."

She got a full ride to Wichita State University. Almost exactly ten years behind schedule, the Bird was finally starting *her* life, pursuing her dream of becoming a teacher.

She had to work full-time throughout. Her boss made her fry the doughnuts every morning at 5 a.m., even when she was pregnant. It made her throw up; that's why he made her do it. Within an hour of getting home from work, she'd be seated at her desk, reading beneath her green-and-gold legal lamp. It could be Shakespeare or Zora Neale

Hurston or John Updike, but whatever it was, it was getting her a page closer to her bachelor's degree in English literature. She finished in four years, magna cum laude.

She was turning her life around but, unfortunately, still not exercising great judgment in the man department. She didn't speak ill of our dad to us back then, though there would have been plenty to say: he didn't pay child support, he was ripsnorting the shit out of some cocaine, he wasn't working, and, perhaps worst of all, he thought he was going to become a famous producer when he moved to Hollywood.

Still, the Bird choosing Mack might've been more forgivable than the man she settled on next—she was, after all, thirteen when she and my dad started dating. They were children. By the time Clyde Nerlinger showed up—about a year after the divorce—she had lived some life.

Alexa knew he was bullshit from the jump. She met Clyde when he came to pick up the Bird for their first date. Alexa was practicing scales on her violin when he knocked. We didn't even know the Bird had a date planned that night, but when Alexa opened the door, Clyde snapped off a formal salute, like a Marine addressing his commanding officer. "Howdy! I'm here to pick up your mother!" He wore a purple satin bowling-team-style jacket with his name embroidered in gold cursive on one breast and a patch that read WAM! over the Chrysler symbol on the other: Wichita Area Mopar Car Club. Parked in our dirt driveway was his membership credentials: a mid-seventies Dodge Charger, bitchin' cherry-red, pretty good condition. That car foretold a future of countless requests to "just drop us off here." We didn't want that thing anywhere near our school. *Holy shit,* my sister thought, *I hope she doesn't marry him.*

"Partner!" he greeted me in a clearly put-on folksy drawl as he brushed by Alexa. He smelled like musky cologne and his jeans were acid-washed and too tight. Also, he had a legit mullet. But I was fixated on that jacket. On the one hand, I couldn't judge his style too harshly. I too owned a satin bowling-team-style jacket. Mine showed that I belonged to the Wichita Force Soccer Club, but it was black, not fucking purple. Also, I was seven. My goalie jersey was covered in Puff Paint and said ZAK ATTACK!

Clyde was a recovering alcoholic and drug addict, deeply beholden to the tenets of both Alcoholics and Narcotics Anonymous — a proud and altogether not anonymous "Friend of Bill W." Pa liked that about him; my grandpa had been sober himself three years now and had become heavily involved with "The Program."

A year later, I was the only one to congratulate the Bird when she told us she was planning on marrying Clyde. At that age, I thought that's what you were supposed to say, what a *grown-up* would say. I felt manhood creeping one step closer as the words left my mouth.

"Congratulations." I nearly laid a firm handshake on her. *Cigars? Champagne? Anyone?* My little brother was five; he didn't get it. Alexa was eleven — she cried; she got it.

"When will he be moving in?" I asked politely.

"Next week."

Truth is, by the time the Bird dropped her bombshell, Alexa had already learned the news. In 1991, the first thing an eleven-year-old girl — even a violin-playing, straight-A kiss ass — did right after school was check the answering machine. "This message is for Clyde and Cindy. We are thrilled to inform you that you've been approved to get married at the Rainbow Event during this year's River Fest!"

"Just tell me why?" Alexa cried. I'd never seen this much pepper out of my big sister.

"That's the choice I've made," the Bird said, sounding a little too resigned to her fate.

But I don't have any trouble understanding why she did it: she was divorced with three kids and worked at a grocery store while taking a full class load. In those days we ate a lot of baloney sandwiches. One slice of baloney, two slices of "cheese," Miracle Whip, white bread. In the summer, there was always Kool-Aid in the fridge—preparing a pitcher of purple was the first culinary art I mastered. Packet of purple, one cup of sugar, stir and refrigerate. Generic mac 'n' cheese on the regular, hot dogs, and ramen—lots of ramen—rounded out the staples. There were more groceries in the fridge after payday than there'd been the entire week before. We didn't have enough money, not even close.

And you don't have to be the most perceptive seven-year-old in the world to see that when your mom puts that brown Dillon's apron on every morning and comes home just in time to tuck you in she is exhausted. That where she's just been has taken something out of her. That it was going to be tough to pull the chain dangling from the green glass shade on the legal lamp.

Clyde, a telephone repairman for Southwestern Bell, could transport us into the security of a squarely lower-middle-class lifestyle, and she liked that he too was a single parent who seemed to care a great deal about his daughter and son. The marriage felt almost arranged, with the Bird as both the bride and the one marrying herself off. For the well-being of her children, *He'll do, I guess*. Her kids needed a man in the house.

River Fest is Wichita's white-trash Mardi Gras. The Arkansas River—pronounced "OUR-Kansas" by the locals—isn't much of a river. When the river is low, an elite long jumper could clear it. So it's a somewhat odd focal point for the city's yearly expression of civic pride. Wind Wagon Smith is the festival's official mascot, played by a prominent member of the Wichita Chamber of Commerce—preferably a fat man, late middle-aged, with a white beard. Santa Claus in a Cap'n Crunch costume, basically. It's an elected position. There was rumor that WWS might grace the Bird and Nerlinger's wedding ceremony with his presence; alas, he had to fire the starting pistol for the bathtub races on the other side of the river. No matter — what the wedding lost in his royal absence was more than compensated for by the enthusiasm of the unwashed masses. Shirtless, sunburned men in frayed cutoffs and baseball caps purchased with Big Tobacco loyalty points crushed Busch Lights on the riverbank while they whooped and hollered throughout the ceremony.

Clyde insisted on wearing full traditional Scottish garb to the wedding: a kilt, knee-high socks with the little garters and flags at the top, a boot knife, a frilly pirate shirt, a jacket that would have looked quite smart on a magician or lion tamer, and *a fucking fur pelt*. The Bird did not want him to wear a kilt. She reminded him he didn't even know for sure that he was Scottish, that he'd never *been* to Scotland, and that he'd never met his biological father (from whom the Scottish blood was allegedly passed). It was embarrassing to her but Clyde was a catch, at least relatively speaking given her current circumstances. The Bird wore a frilly ivory-colored number with lacy sleeves that she found at the Salvation Army for $50. She called it "Spanish." Adam and I wore whatever we'd worn to Easter Mass the previous year, certainly purchased on sale from JCPenney. Alexa wore her violin recital dress, which looked like it was made from the fabric of an old lady's couch. Clyde's two kids rounded out our "white-trash, mutated Brady Bunch," as he liked to call it.

The River Festers on the hill were yelling "Get it!" and cheering like the Chiefs were about to win the Super Bowl when the bride and groom sealed their vows with a kiss. Five or six of them tried to form a human tunnel — the kind parents make for five-year-olds to run through before a soccer game — but it never really caught on. There was no reception after the wedding; the Bird sent us off with Granny and Pa for the night, and the two newlyweds hit the Wendy's drive-thru.

*   *   *

There are two ways to approach the role of new stepdad: You can go the friendly route — soft-pedal, build some trust. *Don't worry, I'm not trying to replace your dad.* Or you can seize the opportunity to lead that totalitarian regime you've always dreamed of. *I am your parent! You will respect me!*

Clyde opted for the latter. He immediately instated something he called Heavy Chore Day — aka, Saturday. Like Sunday Mass, attendance was mandatory but HCD lasted much longer. The whole family was up and working by 0800 and the workday lasted eight hours. Duties were segregated between men's work (in the yard) and women's work (in the house). If there were any holdover friends from a Friday night sleepover, they were welcome to stay, "but if you're here, you need to contribute." Our friends quickly learned to request early pickup times.

Clyde's vibe was all drill sergeant. "Police the lawn for anything that ain't grass or dog shit. Shovel the dog shit. After you mow, edge the perimeter." Half the jobs didn't even make sense: "Move this pile of rocks to the other end of the yard. Dig a hole over here, cart the dirt in the wheelbarrow over there and make a dirt hill."

Absolutely no water breaks until he said "Take five for water, boys!" Unsanctioned trips to the spigot were viewed as obvious attempts to lollygag. Clyde never served in the army, but he did start cutting his hair into a high and tight military flattop; the mullet stayed and he usually wore it in a braided rattail.

Even when it was a hundred degrees and humid as all hell outside, we put in eight-hour days. Light snow, windchill below freezing? "Bundle up, boys!" — eight-hour days. And if it was just *too* goddamn cold, we'd join the women in the house; even with the added hands, the workday somehow still stretched to a full eight hours. "It's training for when you're an adult!"

"I could clean all of this faster than you," he liked to say. "Me and your mom could knock it out; it'd actually be much easier. But you wouldn't learn how to do it. This is how you become a man."

Since Adam was just five years old when HCD started, he only had to pick up rocks. I was eight, so I mowed and edged. The yard was full of goathead thorns, which would get stuck in my shoelaces. Rocks would shoot into my shins from the mower.

But the women's work was worse. "Empty all of the dishes out of the cabinets and scrub the inside of the cupboards with warm, soapy water. Shop-Vac the living room! Not vacuum, Shop-Vac!" And laundry—oh, the fucking laundry. I learned that a week's worth of clothes for seven weighs about fifty pounds. When the weather was nice, Clyde insisted that the clothes be hung on the clothesline, even though we had a perfectly good dryer. Also, my stepbrother couldn't properly wipe his own ass; Clyde was still giving him tutorials well past his eleventh birthday. The girls weren't allowed to throw his Hanes briefs away either; after all, we couldn't exactly afford for him to wear a new pair every day. Instead, they had to scrape his caked-on shit into the trash before washing his clothes—thankfully, at the Bird's insistence, in their own private, contaminated load.

The house wasn't even all that dirty to begin with. Monday through Friday (Sunday being the Lord's day) we received our assignments from the CHORE CHART—a matrix Clyde created with the days of the week running across the top and our names, but not his, running vertically down the side. He was exempt because "My job is to pay the bills and put food on the table. If you want to do that, you can get off the CHORE CHART." We couldn't—child labor laws and all—so it was an empty offer.

The most infuriating part of all the housework was that he acted as if there was some voluntary component to it. "Buddy," he'd ask, "would you mind loading the dishwasher after dinner?" If I said "Yeah, kind of. I have homework," he'd say "Buddy, when I ask you to do something, you do it." If I then said "So, it's not really an 'ask' so much as a 'tell,'" he'd say "I am the *man* of the house."

The Bird had been nearing graduation when she married the new "man of the house." In addition to navigating all the expected difficulties of combining two households, she also juggled forty hours a week at Dillon's, a full course load at Wichita State, and student teaching. As soon as she graduated and began working her "dream job"—teaching language arts to seventh graders at the worst middle school in Wichita—the Bird began to fear that she'd made a horrible mistake. Many days she wondered if she'd done the right thing by leaving Dillon's. My mom worked at that grocery store for fifteen years, through three pregnancies, a husband, a divorce, and a new husband. Just before she left, they offered her a management position. She felt stupid for not taking it—maybe Dillon's *was* a good enough job, and she was *good* at it.

She cried every single day after school. Because she loved to read and write, she thought she'd love to teach others how to read and write. Not true. As soon as she started grading her students' journals, she realized she wasn't an English teacher, just a glorified spellchecker. The kids thought she was fun—she planned her lessons around Ricki Lake and let her students play music in the classroom—but she was too nice. And in these early days, her kindness was exploited as weakness. The gangsters were her favorite kids—the Vato Loco Boys, Folks, Sur 13, Bloods, and Crips—but she couldn't teach the eight parts of speech to kids who read at a kindergarten level. She cried because their parents didn't care if they had four or forty unexcused absences; she cried because she knew what black, blue, red, purple, and green bandanas hanging out of a twelve-year-old's back pocket meant; she cried because she knew her kids had cousins in high school who'd been shot and she knew they were two blocks and two years away from the same; she cried because she was terrified of the parents discovering she was a grocery-bagging fraud who lived in a shit house and had to borrow sugar from the neighbors. But mostly she cried because every day felt like starting a new job — a job she felt she didn't know how to do properly, a job that had cost her four years of sleep-deprived hell on earth to land, a job she thought she hated.

Inside the home, with the addition of Clyde and his two kids, her obligations more than doubled. In the mornings, instead of getting three kids off to school by herself, she now had to get five out the door. Plus Clyde. She was up at 5 a.m. to pack seven sack lunches, including a giant Coleman cooler for him. Her new husband slept until the last possible minute, and once he got out of the shower, he'd stand in a towel in their bedroom doorway and ask, "Honey, can you come braid my tail?" Then he'd insist we all circle up and say the Serenity Prayer or an Our Father. He'd lead us into the Lord's Prayer with "Who makes us a family?" To which the seven of us would collectively answer "Our Father, Who Art in Heaven, Hallowed be Thy name..." At the conclusion of the Lord's Prayer, he'd say, "One day at a time. Keep coming back. It works if you work it!" Between Pa and Clyde, I'd heard it enough by the time I was ten that I started to think I might be a recovering alcoholic myself.

They fought about me regularly. The Bird promised to keep a united front and not undermine him — especially not in front of me — but she tended to take my side when controversy arose between us. For instance, Clyde took issue with the number of hair products I owned and the absurd amount of time I spent on my morning hair routine. In those days I was a Suave man through and through — shampoo, conditioner, gel, and hair spray. If I'd showered the night before, I used a spray bottle to soak my hair from brow to neck. This required a towel to be wrapped around my collar to keep from soaking my shirt. (I couldn't undergo the procedure topless since pulling my shirt on afterward risked ruining the perfection

I had labored so diligently to achieve.) I used a fine-tooth black comb that had been handed out by the good folks at Lifetouch photography on picture day. Once I was good and spritzed up, I would slick back my jet-black hair. It was always tempting to stop there — who doesn't like a good ol' fashioned slick back? But that's a bold move, requiring a certain panache few eleven-year-olds possess; it's a villainous look, best worn by switchblade-carrying street toughs. My favorite shirts featured either Disney characters or soccer — ideally both.

After the slick back, it took eight to ten minutes to find the perfect part on the left side of my head, making sure not a single strand trespassed to the wrong side of the part. Then the final touch: the Swoop. I'd hold my comb parallel to my hairline and run it backward as if I was going to slick back again, but at the last second I'd take a sharp turn off to the right. It's a flick of the wrist, really, and it's this last bit of flair that separates good from great. Finally, I'd preserve my work with twenty to thirty seconds of continuous hair spray. Voilà!

"Do you want him to turn into a faggot?" was Clyde's near daily refrain to my mother. "He uses more shit in his hair than the girls. And he fucking cries if he 'messes it up.'" That all *was* true. My shit was windproof. And I did occasionally cry. I also carried the Lifetouch comb with me just in case the do needed a freshening up after recess soccer. I let the comb peek out of the back pocket of my jeans a bit too — seemed like the right thing to do.

"He cares about how he looks; that's okay," she'd tell him.

My hair was a huge point of pride for the Bird. I was her "Beautiful Black-Headed Baby Boy Born in February" before I was the Gorilla. B.B.H.B.B.B.I.F. "I always wanted a beautiful black-headed baby boy born in February," she told me every February 9. I never questioned the absurdity of wanting such an oddly specific amalgamation of traits. *Ma'am, would you take a beautiful black-headed baby boy born in March? We also have a nice January model available. We could offer you a February, but I'm afraid his hair is just very, very dark brown.*

Another epic battle was fought over the Breyers ice cream that Clyde loved so much. When he discovered that in my twelfth year *I too* had cultivated an appreciation for Breyers mint chocolate chip ice cream, he reacted as if I'd found a way to siphon off his pension and bleed him dry.

"Seems like I had more ice cream than this," he said one evening, genuinely perplexed.

"That's 'cause I ate some," I told him, completely unaware that I was walking into a bear trap.

"You ate some?"

"I did."

"When?"

"After school."

"When after school?"

"Uh, right after school?"

"What day?"

"Hm, every day? Most days? No, every day. Pretty much every day."

"You are eating *my* ice cream every day after school?"

"I'm eating the ice cream that's in the freezer every day after school, yes."

"The Breyers?"

"Do we have another one? Yup, the Breyers."

"That's not acceptable. We're going to have to get you a different ice cream."

I didn't really think about the exchange again until a few days later, when a gallon of Dillon's-brand mint chocolate chip appeared in the freezer, placed in *front* of the Breyers. If the placement of the block-shaped carton was too subtle, there was a note written in Sharpie taped to the lid: FAMILY. And just to remove any lingering ambiguity, on the Breyers: CLYDE ONLY.

I went for the Breyers.

When he got home that night, he went straight to the freezer and saw that neither the high-end Breyers nor the generic cube were still wearing their new signs. This did not sit well.

"Buddy, can you come here a minute?"

I was in the living room, looking over a little algebra, pretending not to hear him. Nestled in my lap: a cereal bowl coated with a few melted drops of white ice cream.

"Buddy? Come in here! I need to speak with you."

I continued to pretend to solve for *y*. *You're gonna have to walk over here, motherfucker.*

"Did you eat the Breyers?"

"*The* Breyers? Like, *all* of it?"

"What's that in the bowl?"

"Mostly nothing."

"What *was* in the bowl?"

"Might have been some ice cream."

"It was the Breyers!"

"How did you know that, because it's not artificial mint-green colored?"

"Did you see the sign on the ice cream, goddammit?!"

"The signs that said 'Family' and 'Clyde Only' in black Sharpie?"

"*YES!*"

"Yeah, saw them. Did you write that?"

"Who the fuck do you think wrote that?"

"A very selfish person, I guess."

"You are not to eat the Breyers!"

By the time I entered high school, tensions between Clyde and me had reached an untenable level. I noticed my friends' parents weren't bitter and resentful. No one else had Heavy Chore Day. The food in their pantries was fair game for everyone to eat. Their parents seemed proud that they played sports, whereas Clyde seemed to view me as the ghost of bullies past just because I was athletic. "Old age and treachery will always overcome youth and skill" was a favorite non sequitur of his. (I'm still not sure what that means.) We'd go days without talking to each other. I tried to set records — fifteen days was as far as I got before I really needed him to pass the salt.

I wanted him to hit me and egged him on at every opportunity. I knew that would end it. And I was pretty sure he'd be up for it. He once told the Bird, "The only thing keeping me from taking that boy into the yard and stomping him is you." The Bird told him, "If you ever touch him, I will have you arrested, but before I do, I will sew you into your bedsheets and beat you with a cast-iron skillet."

By then she knew we needed out, but she didn't know the exit strategy. Money was tight with two incomes. Could we really go back to one? By the end of my freshman year things hadn't been good between them for a few years. I was always the main point of tension.

Finally, he made it easy for her. I'd just come home from soccer practice and was exhausted and starving. He was in the TV room watching *Star Trek*, sitting on his ass, eating Breyers. Didn't even bother with a hello before he said, "Buddy, need you to unload and load the dishwasher. You didn't do it this morning."

"Fuck you! But seriously, fuck you!"

Now he was off his ass — he came at me quick enough that I was sure it was going there, to the yard.

"Go ahead, big boy. Go ahead if you can do it! Fuck me!" He turned around, stuck his big ass into me. "It would be a two-hit fight! I'd hit you and you'd hit the ground!"

I very much did want to go to the yard, wanted nothing more than to be able to beat his ass, but I was about twenty pounds short of capable. He grabbed me just below my shoulders and pinned my arms to my sides. "Old age and treachery will always overcome youth and skill!"

Maybe it was the direct threat of violence, or that he threw the cat off the porch and broke its leg, or that he told my mom she should consider joining a gym and looking up the calorie counts in our meals, or *When you call this house, you need to say, "Hi, this is State Your Name. May I please speak with Zachary?"* or that he plastered the hair from his mullet to the shower wall and made Alexa clean it off, or that he insisted Alexa have her door open at all times, or that he threw the Bird onto the bed and called her a crazy cunt after she told him *Zack doesn't need to ask permission to take a bath in our bathroom,* or the affair, or the accumulation of it all. Hell, maybe it was the fucking Breyers. Either way, we moved out the next day.

On the way out the door, Clyde told her, "You're going to fall flat on your ass without me."

CHAPTER 7

WICHITA (N): TOBACCO, CHEWING TOBACCO, *cigarettes,
Bud Light, Keystone Light, Crown Royal. Muscle-car envy, Camaro,
Chevelle, **Fucked On Race Day**. Join the army. Serve your country.
Church, gun shop, pawnshop. Meth. Baloney, generic cereal, mac 'n'
cheese. Can you lend us a pat a margarine? No shirt, no shoes, no prob-
lem. All you can eat. God hates fags!*

No matter where I'm coming home from, the Wichita-bound flight
is always a puddle jumper with a low ceiling and passengers smiling
like they're boarding the *Titanic*. Officially licensed NCAA and
NASCAR apparel is one uniform. A different uniform is worn by soldiers heading back to McConnell Air Force Base, who are thanked
often and profusely for their service. The earnest, idle chitchat between weary travelers flies fast.

We've got family in Dallas, so we was just visiting.

*Oh yeah? Well, we're going the other way—we have family in
Wichita!*

We are a simple folk.

I was two rows in front of the Bird but I could feel her stank eye
when I ordered my first, then second, then third rum and Coke.

It's only ten minutes door to door from the airport to our house,
and along the way memory lane is paved with Outback, Target,
Pizza Hut Italian Bistro, Village Inn, and the Applebee's where I

went for prom. Before dinner, my date and I took pictures in front of my 1994 Z-28 Camaro and I thought I looked pretty sweet with my frosted blond tips and a diagonal line shaved through one eyebrow. I did not get made fun of for any of that. Pa dropped me $50 for the evening and instructed me to "tell that little girl to get whatever she wants on the menu." That turned out to be the pick-three deal: mozzarella sticks, Bourbon Street Steak, and a Chimicheesecake for dessert. We consummated the special evening at a Holiday Inn Express.

It's a damn near certainty that in any given ten-minute drive in the 'Ta, you will end up at a stoplight with a fella revvin' up a Chevy with a 350 or better under the hood — the unspoken question being *You wanna go?* People are quick off the line, and allowing someone to merge in ahead of you is simply not done. Confederate flags, Calvin and Hobbes pissing on the Ford logo, dangling fake nutsacks, John 3:16, and Kansas City Chiefs arrowheads are the more popular vehicular accoutrements. There was a time when I non-ironically wanted nothing more from life than a full-size K5 Chevy Blazer with thirty-three-inch mud tires, a six-inch lift, and a BIG DICK'S SUSPENSION sticker plastered across the back window.

As we made the left off Ridge Road onto Denmark, our street, I felt a little pang of nostalgia to see the bowling alley at the end of our block. There is something quintessentially Wichita about a packed bowling alley on a Wednesday night. The attached sports bar, Crummie's, hosts nightly karaoke where you can count on hearing an off-key rendition of "I Hope You Dance" followed by a botched "Baby Got Back." There are never more than five audience members, including the three indifferent drunks stuck to their barstools.

I spent my whole life trying to get out of this place. It's as familiar as an identical twin, and yet I still can't wrap my head around the fact that this is the factory where I was assembled.

*   *   *

The Bird's current house on Denmark Street, though far from luxury living, is a huge upgrade from The Palace, where we lived after Clyde. I don't remember packing and we didn't bring much—no bowls, plates, or silverware; a few towels and bedsheets, our beds, the Bird's desk and Gateway computer, a yellow metal folding chair, and the TV. The hulking wood-encased RCA with no remote was worth maybe $50.

Mom didn't tell Granny or Pa that we were moving out until we were gone. Not that there was much time, given that the decision to move and the move itself were separated by fewer than twenty-four hours, but she'd intentionally concealed from her parents how bad her second marriage had become. One divorce was hard enough to own up to.

We needed a new place to live, and we needed it cheap. The Bird was $30,000 in the hole to creditors, soon to file for bankruptcy. The Palace was the best she could do. There was no deposit and there was no first and last. The Bird had a friend who had a friend who was also in need of a housing switch—her husband was getting out of jail and she didn't want to be there when he came back. We took over the $300 rent payment and agreed to store the belongings she didn't have time to pack.

It stank when we walked in. I'd smelled this place before and didn't need to go downstairs to know what the basement looked like: crickets everywhere, wet floor, water-damaged walls, soiled concrete, exposed insulation, galaxies of cobwebs, and a sump pump. Useless for anything but a tornado shelter, and terrifying to children under the age of ten.

The bathroom floor was moist, rotted, and carpeted. When we stepped out of the shower, the floor sunk in several inches. It was clear to all that if we stayed there long enough one of us was going to fall through. Some electrical oddity caused the bathroom sink to shock us every time we turned the faucet on or off. Three of the window-panes were broken, and the backyard looked like a jungle. It would definitely be a loud and painful mow, with sticks shooting into my legs. But at least it would be a voluntary mow—I'd be doing it as a fa-vor to the Bird, not as Clyde's servant.

"Don't think this place is up to code," I told the Bird the day we moved in as we lugged boxes out of the bed of her friend's pickup.

"What are you talking about? This place is a palace," she said.

Granny nearly fell over the first time she saw our new digs. The filth in the kitchen, the musty smell, the heat—she immediately called for a bucket of soapy water and began scrubbing down the cab-inets with a washcloth. Pa was pissed. "Goddamn asshole. Why didn't you call the police and make that sumbitch move out?" He had liked Clyde, but that flipped quick. No AA aphorism was pithy enough to excuse this bullshit. "Seems to me you need a goddamn air condi-tioner," he rightly observed. The Palace was a sweatbox—and it ain't a dry heat in Kansas neither. Pa picked up an old-school window unit—300 or 400 pounds of *real mett-ul* that blasted. "They don't make 'em like this no more. Real mett-ul."

The Palace had two bedrooms, and the Bird gave one each to me, fifteen, and Adam, twelve (Alexa was away at college by then). But the Bird's "room," which was the "office," which was also the "din-ing room," which was also the "living room," was the only one in the house with AC, so from that first night on all of us slept in that one room. The Bird slept on Adam's twin, formerly the bottom half of a bunk bed set he'd shared with our stepbrother. Adam took the blue crushed-velvet couch that the battered woman had left behind. Dust clouds would scatter if you smacked the cushions; he liked it. She had also left an orange pullout, which we christened the meth couch. It looked like it'd been acquired at a police auction after a metham-phetamine den raid. I took the meth couch.

*　　*　　*

My mom started graduate school at Wichita State that fall and once again became a fixture at her desk, the green legal lamp back on every night—busting double shifts again, but at least her day job was no longer sacking groceries. In her second year of teaching the Bird found her stride. She was so good with the "bad kids"—particularly the Vato Loco Boys and other gangbangers—that her classroom became the default destination for students serving "in-school suspension." *Send 'em to McGilvrey* became a popular policy among her colleagues who'd rather not deal with the bullshit.

For the *vatos* that loved to draw, she'd bring in intricate pictures of the Virgin Mary and say, "I bet you can't draw this." After they'd produce some pretty solid replicas, she'd say, "You traced this. I know you did. It's just too good." She started a break-dancing group and an after-school gospel choir. She'd bring in a boom box and big pieces of cardboard for the break-dancers and let them do backflips out of her classroom window. For the gospel singers, Kirk Franklin and the Family albums: "Do you want a revolution?! Woop-woop!"

Her colleagues accused her of making ISS too fun. *It's supposed to be a punishment, you know?* The Bird didn't care. She *loved* the bad kids. Midway through that second year, she figured out why. "It's because I had to raise your stubborn, obstinate ass. They walk slow, cock their chins, trust no one, are viciously loyal to a few. Adults totally write them off, but, thanks to your gorilla coconut-headed ass, I think I get them."

Butch the bulldog—born in a trailer park, purchased for $900 of Clyde Nerlinger's alimony—limped over to me, stiff with arthritis, as I entered the Denmark house through the garage. He head-butted my leg and ran his giant slobbering jowls over the outside of my knee, then snorted with pleasure as I grabbed a handful of excess skin dangling off his face and tugged on the beautiful beast's wrinkled folds.

Over the course of just a few weeks I'd gone from soaring (the co-creator and star of what I assumed would become a hit TV series that would drive me to fame and fortune) to psychotic (parading through the streets of Manhattan in front of imagined television cameras and crew members) to jack shit (back in Wichita, the place I'd spent my whole adult life trying to escape), with no prospects and a mind veering quickly toward the land of depression.

I decided I'd get drunk. What else was there to do? I grabbed the Bird's keys and jumped into her black Dodge Caliber. I missed driving, and the six blocks to the liquor store made a pleasant little field trip. Once I stepped inside, I immediately recognized Mark Hitchcock, an old friend from middle school. Hitch was too smart to be working at a liquor store that sold airplane shooters of Jack by the barrelful. *Fucking Wichita sure knows how to keep a good man down.*

"Hitch, how are you, man?"

He shrugged his shoulders, as if to say *You're looking at it.* But he actually said, "I'm good."

"That's good."

"I saw your mom a while back. She said you're a lawyer in New York? That's awesome."

"Yeah. That's right." I was embarrassed to see him. Neither of us belonged on *either* side of the J&B Liquor counter.

"Better than fucking here. That's for sure."

It seemed like we were both jealous of "my life." I could tell he thought I was sailing in a better boat. I wanted to tell him that it'd sprung a pretty fucking big leak. The Christmas bells on the exit door jingled as I stepped out. I went to the smoke shop next door and bought a pack of Marlboros. It was sweater weather, but there was a guy in a tank top playing Keno. I lit one up in the car and dangled my arm out the window on the way home. Driving while smoking: a great Midwestern pleasure.

The Bird sauntered into the kitchen and eyed my twelve-pack. "Twelve beers, Gorilla? Isn't that a lot of root beers?"

"It might be just enough." I couldn't accurately gauge my own level of sarcasm. "You want to smoke with me?"

"Let me see if I have any menthols."

The Bird is not a smoker, but she normally had a pack of More 100 menthols on hand for when Terry—"my third husband, my fake husband, my best husband"—came over. One pack would last her six months. She and Terry played gin rummy, listened to Al Green, and toked a little weed. The Bird would get buzzed and Terry would get lit. "I got me a fake common-law husband" was her catchphrase on Terry. "Brother won't quit smokin' and drankin' and he's gonna make me a widow." Bird acknowledged that he loved her and marijuana equally, but that was more than enough.

Addiction issues aside, the man had an incredible beard. Solid white, it rose high above his cheekbones. The moustache slightly longer than the rest of the beard and curled upward at the ends. He liked to call himself Black Santa Claus, and he was not wrong. I also knew him to have a nipple ring—the Bird listed it among his assets.

I was initially leery of Terry. Seven years earlier, just a few months after they started dating, he flat-out disappeared for weeks. The Bird was afraid he was dead. She wasn't far off: his brother had died and Terry set out to drink himself into that better place alongside him. When he dragged himself back to the Bird after he'd dried out, she asked me if he was worth another shot. "As long as he's not abusive, it's your call," I told her, knowing she'd take him back. "A dead brother is a pretty good excuse for a bender, but I'll just say 'Fool me once.'"

"By God, shame on you," the Bird said. "I'll just sic my Gorilla on him if he needs an ass whoopin'." She'd need a bigger gorilla if it ever came to that. Terry was a former bodybuilder. He wouldn't even need to put his Newport down to drop me. He drove her crazy with his drinking and smoking—he had a lung condition and a bad ticker from injecting steroids in his twenties, but he still smoked like a stack and put down booze by the 32 oz plastic QuikTrip cup.

Truth was, I was glad the Bird had Terry. And she was crazy about him. Hopelessly in love, really. She loved watching him work our barbecue grill on the weekends; he flipped burgers with his bare hands and refused to use tongs. His grilling outfit was a red bandana underneath a floppy straw hat, and a white cotton tank top. He made his own barbecue sauce, which he kept in a bucket next to the grill and slathered on by the paintbrush. "I love watching that man grill," the Bird would say. Terry would say, "Don't talk to the black man while he's working that grill." Somehow they made that exchange sound nauseatingly sexual. He took the Bird to see plays and jazz shows. They drove out of town for chili cook-offs. She loved that he had decided to go back to school late in life to pursue a degree in psychology. The man thought he'd make a good drug counselor.

And I could tell he cared about my mom. When he showed up post-bender and found out the Bird had gotten a grad student teaching job while getting her PhD at Kansas State, he wept as she revealed her new ID card—the one stamped FACULTY under the picture. "I knew you'd be okay, Cabbage," he told her. Terry would call her at least three times during her two-and-a-half-hour commute to the Kansas State campus. "How's the construction, Cabbage? How many dead deer have you seen? Sit in front and take lots of notes. I'm so proud of you." Terry was no angel, but after what she'd been through with Mack and Clyde, fuck if Terry wasn't all right with me.

I cracked my second beer and stuck my leg out to keep the bully at bay as he tried to head-butt his way into a garage invite.

"When does my brother get home?"

"Tomorrow."

Adam had gone to California to visit our dad.

"Will he ever learn that the well is dry?"

"I hope so."

"I think he still suffers from 'I don't remember living with my dad' syndrome."

"He certainly does. Goddamn Hollywood Peter Pan sperm donor."

The Bird and I enjoy talking shit about Mack. His list of wrongs is not short: the leaving; the utter lack of support; the time he visited me at KU and grabbed some coed's ass in the bar and got us kicked out, then screamed at me the entire walk back to my apartment—"You were on the bouncer's side!" and "Oh, you're so fucking smart, Mr. Lawyer, so fucking smart!"—while kicking me in the back of my foot until I felt it was *imperative* that I punch him in the face. Once I started punching I couldn't stop until I was sure he felt pain. One punch, two punch, three punch. Still not bleeding. I needed him to feel me. I knew thirteen-year-old me was hitting him every bit as much as twenty-one-year-old me.

I picked up my brother from Mid-Continent Airport early the next afternoon. Adam's 220-pound mass shook the car as he plopped down in the passenger seat and fired up a Parliament. His outfit and the longboard strapped to his backpack told me he was back in his skater phase. I took off his L.A. Dodgers hat—new, I assumed—and rubbed my hands through his hair. "Hair looks good; not sure you're going bald after all."

"Fuck you. I'm not."

"You wanna hit up some Applebee's? Chicken tender, riblet pick three?"

"Too fancy, kid."

He wasn't kidding—we'd thought Applebee's was fancy as shit for so long that it still figured in our psyches as a cost-prohibitive slice of luxury.

The lower middle class is precarious territory — it feels closer to lower than middle, and its inhabitants are *allowed* to refer to themselves as "poor" even if they aren't missing meals. We weren't starving; we filled up on Rice-A-Roni. We had shoes and clothes, even brand-name outlet merch at times, but the checkout counter excitement over a new discounted pair of Nikes was accompanied by a stomach-twisting guilt. *Can we really afford these?* Mom or Granny would usually say yes, but there were always pursed lips and deep exhales during the deliberation process. "Okay, but it's your birthday present."

The Bird didn't mind wearing Payless in order to make sure our wardrobes never created a barrier to social acceptance. We wore Payless too, but not a day longer than was acceptable. Once it started to matter, we had the right gear, even if it took a little ingenuity — Alexa wore white canvas shoes from Payless and glued on the blue rubber Keds logo ripped from one of her friend's old pairs. It was tough to see the Bird sacrifice for us, even though she played it off well. "I *like* Payless. It doesn't matter what brands moms wear. Who am I trying to impress?" She could make us believe she preferred cheap, generic shit: "This way I won't care when they get torn up."

Back at the house, my brother tossed his giant skater bag down the stairs and we descended after it into his domain. Adam had just moved back to Wichita and into the Bird's basement after some drug-induced academic troubles at KU in Lawrence. He was trying to wrap up his sixth year of undergrad. On the way downstairs, I surveyed the walls, taking in the laminated Black Jesus picture. There is a wide variety of laminated horseshit in our house; the Bird has a soft spot for any quasi-official document that nods to an academic or employment-related achievement: a Legal Aid business card, for example, or a badge from a teachers' conference. She laminates to "make them look nice." Her signed photo of Alex Haley—author of *Roots*—is displayed between Black Jesus and Terry's last Christmas gift to her: an old lantern affixed to a slab of petrified wood. Terry had slapped a sticker of Jesus on the lantern. I tied my brain in knots trying to imagine how he thought this gift would be received. Had he purchased the Jesus sticker with the intention of decorating the lantern? Had he purchased the lantern at all or did he have it lying around the house already? How long had he known this would be her gift before he handed it over: months, weeks, days, hours, seconds? Was there any internal debate or was he instantly certain that this was just the thing she needed in her life? Did he really think showing up giftless was such a bad idea? Because Terry had laid down a whale of a bet that the Bird landed squarely in the "It's the thought that matters" camp.

The orange shag carpeting starts at the top of the stairs and continues downward and throughout. Fake wood paneling running halfway up the walls enhances the seventies vibe. Since moving back home, my brother had undertaken a few home "improvement" projects piecemeal in the basement. The first to catch my eye: an assortment of hooks drilled directly into the faux wood paneling supporting an equally heterogeneous collection of electric wires, most leading to the far corner, where he'd attached the cable modem to the ceiling with some Velcro straps and a staple gun. It was difficult to imagine any possible aesthetic justification for this new setup.

He'd also installed a "walk-in closet," which he created by knocking a wall down with a sledgehammer so that his formerly closed bedroom now opens into the tiny basement bathroom. A general contractor would call this modification "structural damage."

"So you're basement rich these days, huh?" No rent, free groceries...

"Dude. Are we gonna talk about how you were just in the fucking psych ward, or what?"

I didn't know what to tell him. He considered me his half father—his only decent male influence at any rate. I taught him how to shave, dress, drink, smoke, and talk to girls.

"You should move to New York with me when I go back. I could help you find an apartment in Brooklyn. Get you the fuck *out of here*."

"Bro, *you* are here right now. On some Uncle Eddie shit."

We are both keenly aware that our genes come with a few shallow land mines—the most dramatic case in point being Uncle Eddie. Growing up, my brother and I had kind of a morbid competition to be—and *not* to be—our uncle. Obviously neither of us wanted to end up where he did—institutionalized for life, home for the holidays and the occasional weekend visit, then dead—but if we could just tone him down a bit, erase the schizophrenia and distill him into the bearded wild man with the badass 1970s swag, chain wallet and long hair, smoking hand-rolleds, running from the law, and blasting Pink Floyd so loud it hurt your soul, then what was left was essentially a rock star minus the musical talent.

There were things about Uncle Eddie we both emulated while trying to avoid getting the impression too spot-on. My brother latched on to the druggie part. By age eleven, he was smoking weed every day, then a little coke, then freebasing coke, weed 24-7, alcohol by the bottle in college, more coke, pills. Before I lived in New York, pot was never really my thing, but I have always liked my booze. And, like Uncle Eddie, I've had my nose broken multiple times and run—successfully and unsuccessfully—from the cops on a few occasions.

My mom used to tell us about how Uncle Eddie would eat ice cream so fast that it gave him horrible ice cream headaches, but when Granny would tell him "Slow down, son!" he'd say "I can't! I can't!" and just keep shoveling it in. She said he looked possessed. My ice cream analog was banging my head on the wall and crying for up to an hour about the prospect of dying, starting at age four. "Granny's old—she's gonna die! Then you're gonna die! Then my sissy's gonna die! I don't want to die!" It happened a lot. That scared the Bird. She'd started researching early signs of schizophrenia when I was still in diapers.

Adam started pounding his drums, so I retreated upstairs to watch a little TV. On *SportsCenter,* Tiger Woods either made or missed a putt in China and LeBron James scored a lot of points against the Wizards. There was something funny about the feed, though; it wasn't talking *to* me per se, but it was *maybe* trying to tell me something. The channels weren't changing quickly enough when I hit the button. And the highlights seemed to contain subtle sublim- inal messages that summarized my situation: *Yeah, you just missed a big putt like Tiger, but you're LeBron! You're going to be a scoring machine again in no time.* I wasn't sure; I kept testing the remote, changing channels rapidly and paying close attention to how fast the TV responded. But nothing was so definitively out of order that I felt like I needed to tell anyone. *Crazy man thinks TV is giving him messages. Better to sit on this one for the moment.* The Bird hollered at me from the kitchen: "This is the town crier, announcing that it's time for the big grumpy gorilla's psychiatry appointment." The woman keeps the trains running on time.

In the car, as Kanye built to the line "I bought my whole family whips, no Volvos," a black guy *in a VOLVO!* passed us in the right lane. He was laughing his ass off *and* he looked a little bit like Kanye—same goatee and complexion. *Could it fucking be?* It wasn't Kanye—I knew that. But what if, just what if, the Bird was in on this and The Producer was still pulling strings from New York? Maybe they *wanted* me to go to the psych ward but only because they knew I was exhausted from burning the candle at both ends all summer and that I needed help before our pilot could move forward. Maybe it was a test, and now The Producer was telling me *I'm waiting for you.*

You're still going to buy your whole family whips — they just might be Volvos because you're simple 'Ta trash, and that's good enough. Funny.

"Did you see that?" I asked the Bird.

"What?"

"The brother in the Volvo just now? Right as Kanye said the line about Volvos."

"Nope. I'm not paying attention. This is Kanye?"

Is she playing dumb? Inconclusive.

As we continued the short drive across town, I saw one, then two, B-2 bombers fly overhead. It wasn't unusual to see military planes from the air force base in the sky over Wichita, but I'd never seen two in such quick succession. They were headed east, same direction as New York. "Did you see *that* shit?" I asked her.

"What?"

"The fucking bombers! There! You see 'em?"

"Yes, those are bombers, Gorilla. So what?"

"So fuck. Fuck. Fuck. Fuck."

"Jesus, what?"

"Today is 9/11, part two."

"Today is 11/6, part one, isn't it? What do you mean?"

"Did you see the news yesterday? Fort Hood. Terrorist attack on 11/5. Today is 11/6. Flip it over, 9/11. There's going to be another terrorist attack. And those planes are flying east. New York."

"We are — yeah, I said it: we are!" The Bird was singing along with Kanye. Inconclusive.

Inside the waiting room, Fox News blared on the mounted TV. FORT HOOD. JIHAD. HOMELAND SECURITY. MUSLIM. TERROR. AMERICAN SOIL. But I didn't bring up the bombers again. Before I could decide what to say, it was my turn to see the psychiatrist.

We started with a quick rundown of my mood, progression, mental health history, and current symptoms. *Symptoms?* Oh, for example, was I hearing messages on the TV or anything like that? I wasn't ready to say yes and I wasn't ready to say no, so I split the difference. "What do you mean by hearing messages?"

"Do you believe the TV is talking to you, for example?"

"Well…" I paused for a beat. The doctor's expression informed me that the correct answer was definitely *No*. As in, *No, please don't throw me back in the loony bin*. I played it off. "Well, the TV is *talking* to all of us, isn't it? But if you mean do I think it's tailoring its message to me? Then, no, of course not."

She wrote me prescriptions for Depakote and Risperdal, and we were back in the waiting room. There was a sizeable stack of paperwork to complete and follow-up appointments to schedule. The Bird got down on the paperwork and told me, "You look like a low-blood-sugar gorilla. Go get us something to eat." As I pulled out of the hospital parking lot, I switched from iPod to Power 93.9. Greg the Hitman announced that I'd found "Wichita's home for hip-hop and R&B!" Then he played guess who: Jay Z and Kanye. But it was *old* Kanye — "Never Let Me Down." I drove to Spangles through tears, crying and singing along to what was almost certainly an intervention and reassuring message from The Producer: "When it comes to being true, at least true to me. One thing I've found, one thing I've found. Oh no, you'll never let me down." I was still in the game. *Be brave. Get help. I'll never let you down*, he was saying. *But why such an indirect message? Why not just call me and tell me we're still good, that he hasn't given up?*

The girl at the counter was pretty — a little too pretty to be taking burger orders at Spangles. But everything else was business as usual: fry grease smell, large Wichitans huffing burgers and guzzling Oreo shakes. I looked around for additional reassurances that a local R&B station playing Yeezy and Hova meant something more than the fact that local R&B stations tend to play singles from the two hottest rappers on earth. None came — the pretty Spangles girl tried to upsell me a larger combo and tack on a strawberry shake for only $1 more.

Never before or since have I cried my way both into and out of a Spangles parking lot.

I couldn't make heads or tails of this thing. Is this what hearing voices was like? Maybe when schizophrenics "hear voices" it doesn't mean they literally hear the voice of God or Fat Albert telling them to stab an infant or murder their son on the top of a mountain. Maybe it means they "hear" all the "voices" that are present in the world — songs on the radio, talking heads on the TV, customers in the Spangles express line — and they just make a mess of them.

Later that evening, once the Bird had packed it in, I took a survey of the fridge; since starting back on my meds, I was constantly starving. Hell, yes: hot dogs, ketchup, 2 percent milk, Nesquik, Dillon's sour cream and chive dip, baloney, and some leftover *sopa* from my grandma's house. In the cabinet: Cheerios, Lay's potato chips, white bread. I was staring down a white-trash madeleine de Proust. I wrapped a slice of white bread around two hot dogs and put the bundle in the microwave. While I waited, I threw one slice of baloney down the hatch and grabbed a Kansas Jayhawk coffee cup for the Nesquik. I garnished my hot dog plate with chips and dip and saved the *sopa* — best for last — for round two.

Fishing for a big spoon for my Nesquik and bowl of Cheerios, I pulled open the silverware drawer and froze. The first night I'd spent in Bellevue, fully convinced I was on a disguised soundstage, I'd opened the top drawer of the small wooden dresser next to my bed and heard a nearly onomatopoeic creak. *Creeaaaak.* Slow and spooky, it sounded like a creaky dresser would sound in a movie; that is, perfect — but nothing like a real-life creaky dresser. I was hearing the sounds that we've artificially assigned to certain actions, movements, or objects — like how a bare-knuckle punch in a movie sounds like a mic'd up Mike Tyson knockout blow. I'd laughed at the Bellevue drawer because it was unexpected, but of course that's what it *should* sound like; we were on a soundstage, after all.

The silverware drawer in the Bird's house, however, was not on a soundstage. And yet it sounded just like the dresser at Bellevue. I probably could have tolerated the sound if not for what was inside: a serrated steak knife with a scratched-up wooden handle. It looked like a murder weapon. More specifically, it looked like something Bill the Butcher, Daniel Day-Lewis's character in *Gangs of New York,* might bury into his adversary's ribs. I turned the knife over in my hand and set it down in front of my plate on the kitchen table. *Wait a second,* I thought, staring at the blade. *Aren't all of our knives shitty old knives like this? I've cut a hot dog with you before.*

I went downstairs in search of something I couldn't mistake for a message or a symbol or a planted artifact: my brother. His bedroom is in the back of the basement, a solid forty feet from the stairs, but I could still hear his grizzly snore from the steps. I stood over him in his bedroom and watched him sleep for a minute or two until he sensed my presence and woke up. "What's up, man?" He was groggy enough that he didn't startle.

"Nothing."

"Nothing. You're just standing over me watching me sleep?"

"Yeah, sorry. I was scared."

"It's okay. You need something?"

"Can I lay down for a second?"

"Sure."

He smelled like himself. But his face looked puffier than usual. Fleshy but in an artificial way, like it was made of rubber. "You're *you,* right?" I asked.

"What the fuck does that mean? Yeah, I'm me."

I grabbed his face.

"What the fuck are you doing, dude?"

"I just had to touch your face. To make sure it was you. Sorry." His stubble reassured me. His whiskers were sandpaper-ish but not as thick as mine.

"Sorry. I'm just struggling, man."

"It's okay. You know, sometimes when I'm alone too long I feel like I'm seeing shit that's not there too. Go to sleep, okay?" I dozed off next to him for a few hours before relocating to the meth couch — the freebie from The Palace had made the move with us. The meth couch was authentic, I decided; can't fake the meth couch.

CHAPTER 8

IN THE MORNING, I had to convince myself that, no, there weren't Lollipop kids in the garage, as Lollipop kids were fictitious characters from *The Wizard of Oz*. It was just a coincidence that the red Suburban that drove down our quiet street when I stepped out of the garage was the same model as the one my friend's mom drove in the early nineties. The old people puttering down the sidewalk could look funny unintentionally and effortlessly; no one had to plant them there. Old people *do* look funny.

I took a deep breath and headed over to Granny and Pa's. I have to check in with them within twenty-four hours of landing and I go over to their place every day when I'm in town.

Before he went to rehab, Pa's garage always smelled like Miller Lite, owing to the fifty-five-gallon Rubbermaid trash barrel filled to the brim with empties he can-crushed into hockey pucks. Pa'd jumped at the chance to take Boeing up on their offer of early retirement. "My plan was to just drink. Drink and maybe fish. Sounded like a pretty good plan." Granny finally put a cork in his plan when she found him passed out on the back porch in the middle of February with his head split open. The next day, he asked her, "Are you going to check me in?" Granny said no, she wanted him to do it himself.

I was five when I visited him in the hospital and the nurse told me, "Your grandpa is in the hospital because he is going to quit drinking."

I laughed at her assertion and said, "Yeah, right. All my grandpa does is drink beer, drink beer, drink beer!"

The Bird hit me on the head and told me to cut it out.

Pa took step nine seriously: *Wherever possible, make direct restitution to all persons you have harmed.* He'd been a shit father to the Bird, but he used his grandkids as an opportunity to make it up to her. He told her that she belonged in school, that she must take it when she got her scholarship, and that he and Granny would do anything she needed for her and the kids, financially and otherwise, so that she could finish. We spent most mornings and afternoons after school at their place. Pa was different, no longer grumpy and to be avoided. He hung a basketball hoop in his driveway and taught me how to play H-O-R-S-E. Without them, I wouldn't have been able to play soccer, Alexa wouldn't have been able to take violin lessons, and Adam wouldn't have owned a drum set. I barely remember the North American grizzly. To me, Pa has almost always been a honey bear. Our biggest conflict was usually who would get the gravy first at Sunday dinner.

While I love them both deeply, Granny and I have an extra-special bond. My mom went into labor with me the evening of February 8, 1983. The labor was sixteen hours long and intense. My mom refused drugs and wouldn't consider a C-section. When the Bird was certain it was time to go to the hospital, my dad had carefully rolled and leisurely smoked a joint. She wasn't even all that mad; a joint on the way out the door was par for the course. She was angrier later when, after she'd endured hours of excruciating pain, he left for another quick toke. The man returned to the delivery room and started blowing dank gusts into my mom's face in an ill-timed gesture of assistance. "Breathe, breathe, breathe."

Granny didn't make it to the hospital until hour thirteen of labor. Independent of the birthing difficulties, it'd already been a bad day. All afternoon she'd waited at home for the white coats to come and pick up her son. To Granny, I was his replacement.

*   *   *

Fifteen years later, I had to tell my mom that her brother had died. Granny was crying so hard when she called me that I didn't recognize her voice.

"Granny? What's wrong?"

"King Edward," she said.

"King Edward what?" I knew.

"King Edward is dead!"

"What do you want me to do? You want me to come over?"

"No. No. Not yet. Where's Mama?"

"At school. She has a teacher conference."

"Will you go tell her?"

"Of course."

"Okay, thank you, son." She said thank you. Her cries were primal, but she said thank you.

"We'll be over in thirty."

My car was always Edward's favorite car; that was the only reason it was still in the family. Every time Pa drove to Topeka to pick him up for a visit, Edward had two requests: first, "Bring the piss cutter"; second, "We're going to Godfather's and I'm eating a whole goddamn pizza." A 1974 Dodge Dart Swinger, 318 engine, white hardtop. It *was* a fucking piss cutter. I shouldn't have been allowed to drive it — way too much car for a fifteen-year-old.

John Marshall Middle School was four minutes away if you followed the speed limit. My aim was to get there in under two. Anything slower felt like an affront to Uncle Eddie, not only because this news was so awful it demanded to be relayed instantly but also because he was so newly dead that it almost felt like his spirit was still fresh enough that he might be able to feel that piss cutter roar one more time. I J-turned out of the driveway and proceeded to cut piss.

In two blocks, I had her up to eighty. In three more, I'd need to stop and make a right turn. Before I got there, a woman in a Buick LeSabre failed to recognize that I was doing four times the speed limit and thought she could make a lazy left turn out in front of me. The piss cutter was rear-wheel drive, of course, and she locked up immediately. My back end fishtailed left, then hooked right, and I exploded into the curb. It was a one-car accident, but I hit the curb so hard that I felt lucky I didn't go through the windshield.

The cops were there quickly; I assume the crash was loud enough that a neighbor called them. That or the yelling.

I was still yelling "Fuck!" when the first cop pulled up. Of course everyone assumed it was about the car.

"I have to get out of here! I have to go!"

He must have been among the most reasonable officers in the world, because if not, I'd have been on the ground. It was my fault, I was flipping out, and there was a middle-aged white woman pointing a finger at me.

"My uncle is dead! My uncle is dead! I'm going to tell my mom! She's at Marshall! She's a teacher at Marshall!"

Paperwork was filled out, and soon enough I was dropped off in a squad car at the Bird's school.

I went to the library on the second floor. The place smelled like seventh grade and Coach Nash, but I'd never felt more like a grown-up in my life than when I walked into the library. I wasn't crying—tried to poker-face it—but before I could ask anyone if I could steal Ms. McGilvrey away, the Bird was out of her seat. I made a head nod toward the hall.

"What did you do?" She was frantic.

"King Edward."

She knew, just as I had known when Granny told me, but she made me say it.

Middle school hallways echo loudly. I could see the other teachers through the library's portal window. Her screams left no doubt that someone had died. They'd have come running otherwise. I made eye contact with Mrs. Farley, my algebra teacher, and motioned that we were leaving.

I practically carried her downstairs and to her car.

Even though I hate it when Granny smells smoke on me, I smoked two cigs as I made the drive over for our morning routine. Eggs, bacon, *Wichita Eagle,* twelve o'clock news. Pa was eating his grapefruit at the bar when I walked in through the kitchen door. Granny was ironing in the basement, blasting Pink Floyd. You wouldn't know it by looking at her, but the eighty-year-old with the beehive hairdo worships at the altar of Mick Jagger, Jimi Hendrix, and Roger Waters. She fell in love with the soundtrack to her son's hell-raising days and she's been ironing to acid rock ever since. Her perfect day starts with a load of clothes in the washer and the Stones or Floyd on the radio. Her dryer is fifty years old and weighs half a ton, but it still works as well as the day the Maytag man delivered it — probably because it doesn't get much work. If it's over thirty-five degrees outside, the dryer gets the day off and our laundry is pinned on the clothesline. Then she irons. Everything.

While it's nice to have someone willing to wash every stitch of the entire family's soiled clothing, the favor does come with a price. First, you load up forty or so pounds of laundry in various old bags that are not fit to serve as a carry-on — old denim Winnie-the-Pooh gym bag with a missing strap, for example — and drive them to her house. You throw the giant sacks and bags and hampers down the basement stairs. Imperative: do *not* forget to leave explicit instructions not to iron T-shirts, jeans, or underwear. "Not even the jeans? Just a little touch-up? Just a touch-up, son. Please." Omit that warning, and your jeans will be returned heavily starched with a razor-straight line running down the middle, Granny pleading innocence all along: "Oh, you didn't say no crease, did you?" Depriving her of the pleasure she gets from putting a firm press on a pair of Levi's feels almost sadistic. But I make it up to her by letting her feed me a lumberjack's breakfast every morning when I'm in town.

Granny rushed up the stairs, gave me a half hug, and took my and Pa's orders: bacon, eggs; no toast; okay, juice if you insist; yes, coffee. "Can I talk you into a tortilla on the *placa?*" The *placa* is a heavy, plate-shaped iron artifact from the farm where she grew up in Tonkawa, Oklahoma, that she uses to heat up tortillas with melted cheese. Granny thinks she's Mexican—and she's at least half—but she also never met her mother, who may have been Native American. She looks more Lebanese than anything, but she rolls her *r*'s when she pronounces "Doritos." *Dorrrritos.* I agreed to the tortilla on the *placa.*

Pa treats being waited on hand and foot as a huge burden that he somehow overcomes. "William! Are you ready for breakfast?!" For years he's claimed to have "selective hearing" but it's now undeniable that he can't hear much—Granny shouts everything at him. "William! Do you want sausage or bacon!? Turkey bacon or regular bacon!? Oatmeal!?" "Did you wash up, William?!"

He buried his head in his hands as Granny rattled off the day's specials. "Help me, dear Lord. Help me accept the things I cannot change. This woman."

"Pa, it must be awful having someone who lives to serve you, does all the cleaning and laundry, and cooks whatever you want for your every meal," I teased him.

"Weezy's a pretty good ol' gal," he said as she clucked and sucked her teeth.

"Mm. That man. I swear." It's quite an act.

Over breakfast, I read the *Wichita Eagle,* or at least what was left of it. Wichita's paper of record felt like a pamphlet; it was down to four or five pages. My favorite is the Opinion Line: "Obama still has not produced a birth certificate." "We need to have mandatory drug testing for welfare recipients." "Liberals want to take away the Second Amendment, but they can pry my guns from my dead, lifeless fingers." "God made Adam and Eve, not Adam and Steve."

After breakfast, Granny finishes the dishes and it's over to the couch for the twelve o'clock news, which is basically a recap of the previous evening's five and six o'clock programs. I usually doze off halfway through the newscast. Pa sleeps in his chair. Neither of us is allowed to touch the dishes.

He falls asleep at the slightest lapse in conversation, but he's not offended if anyone does the same, even if he's in the middle of one of his stories. I know them all verbatim. "We once went out and got pretty tuned up, and old Captain Bobby knew about it. He got our asses out of bed at six in the morning and took us on a full-pack, twenty-mile field march." Or "Madre's father was a tough ol' S.O.B. He was an old farmer — that's the way they had to be." Or "I went to New York one time. We were staying in Danbury, Connecticut. We drove into the city and tried to go to TGI Fridays, but we couldn't find it so we went back to Danbury." There are a few more in the regular rotation — one about how when he was in "Ki'rea" the "Ki'reans respected us for our arms and we respected them for their legs. They had powerful kicks." Another concerning how there really is no such thing as friendly fire. Also, never forget that the number one thing to do with your car is to "make sure there's 'erl in it — good rubber is important too."

It was depressing to be there, watching Pa grow increasingly frail and more and more dependent on Granny to get through his day. And Granny, while still stout as a mule and sharp enough to espouse passionate opinions on the artistic merits of Lady Gaga and Miley Cyrus versus Taylor Swift — loves the former two, loathes the latter — no longer possesses the stamina she did in her seventh decade. Their house has always been a sanctuary for me. I spent countless grade school mornings getting ready for school and eating Cheerios and eggs at that breakfast bar before Granny dropped me off at school; an equal number of evenings sleeping with Adam and Alexa on pallets of blankets on the floor before the Bird could pick us up at the end of her grocery store shift. In high school, before I could drive, it was six eggs and six pieces of bacon after soccer practice. Now, with their mortality front and center, I wanted to spend as many hours as I could with them. But I also wanted to flee after breakfast.

Most days I made it through at least the five o'clock news and checked out before sports in the middle of the six o'clock rerun. Between the paper and the two and a half local broadcasts, I stayed pretty well informed on Wichita current events, hanging out with Granny and Pa. On my way out the door, Granny would laugh while piling hangers of ironed gym shorts onto my fingers. "I'm going to load you down like a burro, Zachariah."

My evening routine was as formulaic as my afternoon with the old folks. Garage. Beer, smoke. Beer, smoke. Sit in the kitchen, stare at bulldog. Garage. Beer, smoke, smoke, smoke. How many cigarettes can I smoke in a row? Four or five spread out over three beers felt about right. Then two more. Around beer six, I'd start thinking, *Okay, two or three more, then let's call it.*

Remnants of high school are jammed into the back corner of the garage: a stack of goalie gloves, Northwest Grizzlies posters the cheerleaders made when we went to State, a thirty-six-inch plyometric box turned upside down — inside that box, several pairs of soccer shoes, a jump rope, a weight vest for running wind sprints. Relics that used to define me. It was hard to believe that I once used peroxide to dye my black hair blond in a show of team solidarity; or that we used to hold freshmen down and slap their bare bellies until they bled; or that I'd been proud to be one of only two players my freshman year to *receive* a red belly; or that I had a letterman's jacket on order before they even handed out the patches. The boy who wore military fatigues on game day had become a different person.

But who?

Ever since my stepdad started calling us poor white trash when I was eight years old, I became obsessed with proving him wrong. *Speak for your damn self, buddy. My mom goes to college and we all make straight A's. I play soccer, my sister plays the violin, and Adam will do something too when he gets bigger. You're the one with a flattop and a mullet that you braid into a rattail. You're the one who barely graduated high school. You're the one who goes to the Taco Tico and orders "just a cup o' meat, partner."*

I was proud that the boy who'd once been called a faggot for styling his hair in the 'Ta went on to live with gay guys in Brooklyn. Hell, just not being racist felt like an accomplishment at a certain point in my life. I never imagined I'd someday have heated discussions about transgender rights or know what "cis" meant. But where was all that now? I was living in the goddamn garage. A week earlier I'd been involuntarily committed to a psych ward. Mr. Fucking Lawyer. Sure as my brother was in the basement snorting Addies, I was staring at the NORTHWEST GRIZZLY WINNING FORMULA, kicking a flat soccer ball against the wall, so tipsy I could barely make contact, and drinking the same cheap beer we shotgunned after games. Good job not thinking it's awesome to wear camo cargo pants anymore. Good job getting over subwoofer envy. Good job not getting in a fight for a couple of years. But fuck — what's a JD worth in the fucking garage? Pretty good résumé you've got there, bub. Overqualified for making ash heaps on top of Coors Light cans.

The Bird popped her head in the garage and did a few head rotations. "Just a reminder for the gorilla in the lawn chair surrounded by beer cans and smoking like a trucker: you have your second psych appointment tomorrow."

"Appreciate it. Night."

"The town crier will be sounding her trumpet at nine a.m."

*　　*　　*

The teenager sitting across from me at the Via Christi Behavioral Health Center annex was wearing huge wide-legged jeans and a black wolf T-shirt with purple and white lightning bolts shooting down from the moon behind the wolf's head. He looked like he was no stranger to a Mountain Dew for breakfast. I imagined we were looking at an oxy addiction, maybe meth too. His mom sat next to him, purse lipped and scowling before muttering something about "Last time, goddammit. Last chance, mister. Ya understand?"

He reminded me of the kids that lived next door to us growing up. The ones that smelled like piss and child abuse. Shirtless in February and covered in dirt and Kool-Aid and screaming at us to stay off their fucking property—when they were *six* and *four*. And the Bird used to have to borrow margarine from *them*.

A medical assistant walked out dressed in sea-foam-green scrub bottoms and a white top covered with teddy bears holding balloons. She had straight bangs, a wet perm, and a yellow dye job. "Zachary McDermott, the doctor is ready for you."

The psychiatrist, a middle-aged African American man, was jacked. I wondered if he worked out at the West Wichita YMCA or Gold's on Central. As he started to ask questions, I pictured him bench-pressing 350 pounds while his lifting partner stood over him and screamed *Lock it out, bro!* There was a framed copy of the Serenity Prayer on the wall.

He started the interview in a doctorly monotone.

"How is your mood?" he asked.

"I don't have a mood."

"What do you mean?"

"I mean I can't feel anything. Nothing. I'm not here."

"Every drug has side effects."

"I hear that. But—and I'm just going to lay this out here in the interest of time—my hair is falling out. I'm drooling. I'm impotent. I can't ejaculate. I go minutes without even realizing I'm awake. And I've gained ten pounds in a week."

"The sexual side effects—the libido, the impotence—are common with Risperdal. As is weight gain, but that's primarily coming from the Depakote."

I knew where it was coming from; I just wanted to know where we go from here. "So what's the solution?"

"In three or four months we can maybe reevaluate."

"Three or four months? And reevaluate? Maybe? I can't be impotent for three or four months. I'm twenty-six. I know this might not sound like the most important thing, but it's important."

He continued with what felt like a standard questionnaire—much like the one I'd filled out before I entered his office.

"Are you using any drugs—cocaine, marijuana, heroin, methamphetamine?"

"No."

"Drinking alcohol?"

"Yes."

"How much are you drinking?"

"I don't know. Minimum four, more like six beers a night. Sometimes eight, sometimes ten."

"That's a lot."

"Can we get back to that medication for a minute? What happens if I go off it?"

"You can't quit taking it."

"And if I do?"

"Severe depression is almost certain. And you'd be at high risk of having grand mal seizures."

"What are the odds of that realistically happening?"

"I can't tell you that."

"Can't or won't?"

"I cannot."

"Because you don't know or because you have a legal obligation not to tell me so you're not tacitly endorsing the sudden cessation of medication?"

"I can't."

"Well, thanks, that really helps me make a rational decision on this topic."

"Zachary, are you going to quit drinking or not?"

"Certainly not while I'm in Wichita."

That goddamn Serenity Prayer really pissed me off.

Lord, grant me the serenity to accept the things I cannot change,
the courage to change the things I can,
and the wisdom to know the difference. Amen.

Was this supposed to be an "accept the things I cannot change" situation or a "courage to change the things I can" situation? Accept what? Impotence, drooling, a brain firing at half capacity? Yes, I was drinking too fucking much, but my mania was precipitated by insomnia and at least the booze was knocking me out. Binge drinking felt safe. It was the devil I knew.

I did go to one of the substance-abuse meetings the doctor had pushed on me, the following Wednesday night, back at the clinic. The Mountain-Dew-for-breakfast kid was there, along with some folks who reminded me of characters from my first neighborhood: the tweaker who used to blast Whitesnake and rip tits in his Trans Am down our street, the dude with the boa constrictor. So much meth face, including a few that looked to still be tweaking. The guy sitting next to me smelled like my dad's brother, Uncle Randy, who shits in Folgers coffee cans. For a second I thought I really did recognize my friend Colt's sister, who, last

I heard, was stripping at Jezebel's. I thought about leaving—I was still not ready to consider quitting drinking—but I wanted to gawk.

We watched the Michael Keaton movie *Clean and Sober*, where he drinks his life away and then recovers. There was also free pizza. I tried not to eat it at first, as I judged everyone else in the room for being too excited about free junk food. But eventually I caved and ate two slices of pepperoni. If I was going to quit drinking, this wasn't going to be the route. You can't feel superior to everyone in the room and simultaneously address your own problems. And in this room I didn't see people *with* problems; I saw people who *were* problems.

The Bird picked me up. "How was it?"

"Ridiculous. Absurdly white trash. Watched a movie. More than two tongue rings, both sexes. Not going back."

She didn't say anything.

When we got home, I started drinking.

A week later, I quit taking my meds. I couldn't even follow the plot of *30 Rock*, and the Bird had to dab drool off my face several times a day or say "Gorilla, look at your shirt." I'd sit alone in the basement with my hand on my penis and jiggle it around just to see if he had any intent of ever having any intent again. My hair was coming out by the handful in the shower, and I'd put on nearly twenty pounds. I told the Bird I was going to go off the meds before I pulled the plug. She was worried about a lot of things, but seizures were pretty high on her list. She told me, "I am terrified for you to go off your medication. But I see what this is doing to you and I can't tell you not to."

While the seizures never came, the doctor's prediction of severe depression was no joke. I began to have contests with myself to see how many hours I could sleep each day. Getting to twelve without a nap was no problem. With naps I was able to get to fourteen and, occasionally, even sixteen. My days became a countdown to an acceptable sleeping hour. To fill the gap between my final nap and bedtime, I drank and smoked. Beer. Cig. Beer. Cig. Cig. And so on. Now I understood how so many men I'd known growing up could burn through a twelve-pack every night. What else do you do here? People say that excessive drinking is often used as an escape from reality. In my case, I felt erased, so why not erase myself? It was easier to chip away at what was left of me than to try to recover the self I'd lost.

CHAPTER 9

THE BIRD SHOUTED DOWN the stairs when he came in through the garage: "G-O-R-I-L-L-A, your B-R-O-T-H-E-R B-O-B-B-Y is in the kitchen." Bobby had been out of prison a little more than a year and I hadn't seen him in six, but other than a little prison bulk and a hairstyle change from S Curl to shoulder-length braided pigtails, he looked exactly as I remembered him.

"What up, cuz?" Sounded the same too.

I'd been staring at the ceiling, in and out of sleep for several hours.

"You look like a sad old butthole," he told me. We hugged and I told him he was huge.

"*Swole*, cuz," he corrected me.

"Prison swole."

Bobby Prince Jr. was born a Crip in the same way that many Irish boys in Boston are born Catholic. The Bird called him B-O-B-B-Y but he usually corrected her and said "C-O-C-C-Y — Bobby got too many *b*'s, cuz." *B* as in Bloods.

Bobby — two years younger than me — was patient zero at Power Hour, the Bird's informal after-school tutoring group that she started when I was a senior. From the beginning, it was populated exclusively by young black men, each with one gang affiliation or another. Warring factions coexisted peacefully as the Bird fed everyone and tutored two or three kids at once while a handful of others shot hoops in the driveway or lifted weights downstairs.

Bobby's powder-blue 1990 Nissan Maxima was a fixture in our driveway every afternoon. You knew he was coming before his whip came into view because he bumped Lil Wayne or Birdman so hard his trunk shook. The car had plastic hubcaps posing as chrome rims and he was saving up to get a portrait of himself painted on the hood. "Gotta show 'em the grill, cuz." He was proud of the gold outlines on his front teeth, and he pulled off the look.

In those days, Bobby's backpack overflowed with letters from Division I colleges offering him full rides to run track—Arizona, North Carolina, Kansas, Texas, Oklahoma, Clemson, Ohio State, and nearly every school in between—but when he came into our lives, it appeared he had no hope of being able to accept any of them. He was a sophomore in high school, but his ACT score was several standard deviations below the NCAA's minimum requirement and Bobby couldn't read for shit. One reason being, he didn't start going to school until third grade. He struggled to get through Dr. Seuss books for the first few years.

Bobby was born in a trailer in rural Oklahoma, or as he put it, "deep, deep in the country, country." Anywhere between three and six cousins, along with his grandparents, slept together in the main room of a double-wide. There were a couple of other rooms, but they were filled with junk—"like hoarder-type stuff, cuz." They had no electricity, running water, or plumbing. When he had to do his business, it was in The Bucket—which is exactly what it sounds like. Six to nine people pissed and shat in a big white bucket that was kept in the bathroom and emptied not near frequently enough. "When you grow up doing that as a child, you look at things different when you become an adult and actually get to sit on a toilet and shit. I can do my business anywhere. Put some paper down, bro, I'm good. Some people say that's disgusting, but what's disgusting is The Bucket."

Bobby learned pimping from his father when other kids his age were learning their ABCs. After his mom got out of prison, he moved to Kansas to be with her. But in the summers, she'd drop him off with his dad at the Kansas-Oklahoma border. What she didn't know was that she was leaving him at the "Ho House." Bobby Prince Sr. dropped him off with his women while he handled his business. They took him shopping, buying him clothes and Nikes. Before his voice dropped they were asking him, "You trying to get that wooty, B.P. Jr.?"

Power Hour grew fast, thanks to Bobby. Week after week, new faces showed up. Bobby started calling my mom "Moms." The Bird stacked pyramids of cheap beef and generic shredded cheese soft tacos in the fridge. It was by no means decadent, but Bobby always said, "You know Moms can cook." He grew up on SPAM and rice, so the Bird's meals seemed gourmet. One day the Bird overheard him telling a new recruit, "This like a real home, bro. You come home from football, you get food in your belly, and you take care of your school business." He put in hundreds of hours with the Bird; eventually, he could work his way through *Lord of the Flies*. When the Bird explained to him that the character Piggy was tender, he asked her what that meant. "He's vulnerable—asthma, glasses, people always pick on him."

"Oh, I got it," Bobby said. "He a tender booty."

The towels were emptied from the cabinet next to the bathroom and replaced with cheap peanut butter and jelly, bread, canned ham, crackers, Vienna sausages, ramen noodles by the case, and tuna for protein. When word of Power Hour reached Holy Savior—the Bird's predominantly black Catholic church—Alfred Wright, a beloved church elder, brought over fifty-count boxes of frozen corn dogs. Bobby called Mr. Wright "Shoe Booty" behind his back because his left leg was almost a foot shorter than his right, forcing him to wear an enormous platform shoe on one foot. It looked extremely heavy and gave the impression that Mr. Wright's limp stemmed from the difficulty of lifting that damn shoe with every left step.

Once Shoe Booty said hi to all the boys and filled the freezer, he'd often give the Bird $50 or $60 to use as she saw fit on the Power Hour crew. As soon as he was out the door, Bobby would grab a jar of peanut butter from the pantry and put his foot on top of the lid while he herked and jerked across the room, deftly dragging the peanut butter beneath his foot. It was a pretty convincing act, especially given the difficulty of the prop work—he never tipped the peanut butter onto its side, or lifted his foot off the top of the jar.

"What's a corn dog?" Beast—another Power Hour regular—asked.

"Nigga, you know what a corn dog is. Your lips is corn dogs."

Bobby had a full set of lips of his own, but that didn't stop him from holding two frozen corn dogs to his mouth and doing a pretty spot-on Beast impression: "What's a corn dog? Nigga said he don't know what a corn dog is!" He flapped the dogs as he talked. "Here, Beast, I'ma put your lips in this microwave for you." And then he prepared a corn dog for Beast.

After a little more than a year of Bobby coming to Power Hour, he was doing well enough on ACT practice tests that it looked like he might score high enough on test day to accept one of his scholarships. The Bird couldn't sleep the night before his test. She knew Bobby would need to have one of his good days to qualify, and she did a rosary in hopes of giving him a divine edge. Bobby didn't leave his fate to the gods, though.

If he was going to have someone take the test for him, there was only one high school where that'd be conceivably possible: Northeast Magnet. They didn't have an athletics program, and anyone who knew anything about Wichita football, basketball, or track—a good chunk of the Wichita population—would have recognized Bobby Prince. If he was four inches taller he could have played in the NFL. He thought he could score high enough on his own, "but dawg, I had to get that scholarship. You think a kid like me is supposed to go to Arizona? You gotta make sure." And make sure he did. "Bobby" scored six points higher than his best practice score.

An administrator actually tried to get him to admit that he cheated, that he'd paid someone to take the test for him. But Bobby wasn't about to buckle under a threat of fingerprint testing from an assistant high school principal. He told the guy, "Y'all think I'm dumb, and this is starting to feel a little bit racist." They dropped it.

He decided to go to Butler County Community College for a year before transferring to a four-year college so that he could play one more year of football and better prepare himself for "a real school."

He got shot the night of his senior prom.

Bobby had been on the wrong side of town wearing the wrong colors. When he stopped at QuikTrip to get some rubbers, he wasn't too worried about the fact that there were two Bloods in the parking lot staring him down. Being C-O-C-C-Y, he was decked out in a Southpole blue and yellow polo with matching jeans and all-white Reeboks with blue laces. The Bird told him, "You look like you're headed to the Players' Ball," when he stopped by the house to take pictures with his date.

He didn't notice that the red hoodies at the QT followed him to his hotel room. If the shooter hadn't yelled, "What up, Blood?" before squeezing the trigger on his 12-gauge, Bobby would, in all likelihood, be dead. He'd just opened his hotel room door; Bobby threw his date into the room so she wouldn't get hit, but the Blood got him in the shoulder. He didn't know the guy and is pretty sure it was a gang initiation. No one was arrested, but "maybe something happened to him."

The shooting pretty much closed the book on school for Bobby. He told the Bird he was going to move to Oklahoma to be with his daddy. The Bird and Bobby's mom begged him not to go, told him nothing good was down there for him and he could still go to school once he healed. "It ain't forever, Moms. I can be a country nigga." Bobby wanted to get to know his dad.

Six months later, he was standing next to his dad in federal court, entering a guilty plea for his involvement in an interstate truck stop prostitution ring. Bobby Sr. had rolled on his son and told the feds that he had no involvement—that it was all B.P. Jr.'s doing. Bobby took five years and ten months; Senior got double that.

It was all over the papers—even made *People* magazine.

The Bird was at the Urban League Learning Center in the middle of the school day when she heard the news. Her colleague, a 500-pound bigot and football fanatic whom the kids called Shamu, gleefully read the headline to her. "'Former NW Football Star Charged with Sex Trafficking.' What do you think of your Bobby Prince now?" he asked the Bird. She started shaking and weeping and left the room. She was crushed, but also pissed. How could B-O-B-B-Y do that? Why hadn't she tied his ass down and told him she'd only free him after he got the fool-ass Oklahoma idea out of his head? She remembered the day they got "his" ACT score, how they'd jumped up and down together. What was going to happen to B-O-B-B-Y in prison?

"So? How's being out?" I asked Bobby.

"Man, bro. Fucking internet, man. I'ma learn that computer. Is you on Facebook?"

"Barely. I wouldn't learn that first."

"Everybody got they little computer on they phone now. When I went in, people was just starting to fuck with the flips and we thought that was dope. My moms stays on Facebook."

"I stays on Facebook too," the Bird chimed in. "Gets people into the Bird's school. Turning tassels."

"You *do* be turning tassels. *Do*." This is one of my favorite Bobby verbal tics. If you ask him if he has a date: *Do. Do have a date.* Did he hit? *Did hit. Did.* Is his car clean? *Is, cuz. Is clean.*

I shooed the Bird away and told her we had man talk to discuss.

"Do."

"But for real, C-O-C—are you all right? You fucked-up?"

"Man, prison, cuz? You trying to hear 'bout prison?"

"Would. Would hear about prison," I said.

"Tell you the truth, bro. People don't like to talk about prison, mostly. But, shit, I tell you. Watch'u wanna know?"

"Well, the obvious. Anybody get that BPJ wooty?"

"Nigga said 'Anybody get that BPJ wooty?'—what you think, cuz?"

"Hope not."

"Didn't. Did not. Man, it's like this, cuz: I'm a Crip, right? Been a Crip. *Been.* But when I went in, I wan't trying to be 'bout that life. I coulda got in with them—everybody knew me in there. I had fam in there. I had niggas in there that knew my fam. I coulda bunched up, you know? But I just wanted to do my little time, man. And you know me, I ain't got no enemies. I can get along with e'rybody. So I didn't really have no beef with nobody."

"Never? Were you ever scared?"

"Bro, I'm telling you. Prison wasn't all that bad. Moms was writing me. Couldn't never call, 'cause that shit's expensive, cuz. But I just did my little time. I got in one little beef—that was the only time I was scared. But not 'cause I couldn't handle ol' boy, it's just—shit don't end in hands there. Traditionally. *Don't.*"

"Kill him?"

"You know I ain't no killer, bro. Nah, we was playing basketball and I was talking shit—you know how I fuck around. And this dude was younger, so he, I guess, felt like he was being disrespected, but I was just playing. And dude couldn't hold me, and I just kept telling him, 'Bro, you know you ain't gonna guard me. You gotta get somebody out here to guard me.' Ol' boy just kept trying to guard me and I just kept scoring. And so anyway. I could tell he wanted to fight me and I could tell we was going to have to do it there on the yard. 'Cause you ain't trying to get it in the cell, cuz. So anyway, I told him, 'Come on, then, if you need it. If you need it, come get it.'"

"You win?"

"Bro, I ain't trying to be cocky—but you know I can fight. I wasn't even mad, but I think dude just felt like he had to fight me. So, yeah, I touched him up a little bit. And then I hear that ol' boy wants to stab me and I'm like, well, fuck. I got dudes offering to shank him for me, but I ain't trying to hurt nobody. And, man, you know I can talk to people. So I just went up to him and told him, 'Man, I ain't even got no beef like that.'"

"That was it?"

"*Was.* Was it. And that was the last fight I was in. Because, bro, check it. We play basketball in there. And I ain't bragging, I'm just telling you that—"

"You're fast as piss."

"*Am.* And they saw me touch dude up so, man, think about it. They know I'm fast and they know I can fight, so if you trying to look tough and then you get your li'l ol' ass kicked. Bro, it don't work, you know? So I was chilling. But mostly just 'cause I ain't got beef like that with nobody."

"You act like it wasn't all that bad."

"Ain't trying to go back, bro. I seen some horrendous shit. Like, two dudes, one Mexican and one black dude, raping this white dude. Hearing that, bro, I will never forget that sound. I saw dudes get stabbed, they bleeding out. Dudes is playing cards, another nigga bleeding to death. But I *ain't* broke. I got all my limbs and my teeth and my kneecaps."

Listening to Bobby recap the first half of his twenties for me, all I could think was *What a waste of life.* Bobby didn't even know how fucked he was now that he was out, how hard it was going to be for him to ever get a job with health insurance. Six years in prison makes you a convict for life. Bobby was looking for work, but it would take a strong character reference from the Bird just to get him hired in the stockroom at Dillon's after checking the FELON box. His conviction also made him ineligible to receive federal financial aid, so going back to school was out. In all likelihood, because of some admittedly fucked-up stuff he did when he was eighteen years old, he'd peaked at prom king.

I had written my law school application essay about the atrocity of Bobby's life and imprisonment. Here he was, personal statement in the flesh, calling me out. I couldn't remember the exact wording, but I was pretty sure my essay mentioned something about how I was determined to dedicate my life to defending those whom our society was failing and the criminal justice system was destroying. As best as I could recall, it didn't say anything about sitting on a lawn chair in my mother's garage, crushing eight domestic beers every night.

Most people, even most liberals, don't give much thought to the fate of guys like Bobby. They subscribe to the good/bad binary and, to them, Bobby is a no-brainer bad dude, guilty of participating in an interstate truck stop prostitution ring. It's easy — and convenient — to believe that jail is an acceptable solution to the question of *What do we do with all of these felons, most of whom seem to be black?* No part of the criminal sentencing process asks: "Was his dad a pimp or an accountant? Did his dad encourage him to join the family business? Is locking him up going to do anything for him or us in the long run? To what extent was he just a cog in a larger machine in which he had no free will?" These sorts of considerations confuse the narrative: only bad people commit crimes, and it is okay to put bad people in cages. Easier not to think too hard on it.

On top of that, had Bobby been caught a few months earlier, the courts would have chalked up his crimes to his undeveloped adolescent brain. Magically, on his eighteenth birthday, he transitioned from wayward youth to evil man. So we slapped him with 2,190 days in federal prison instead of probation and an expungement. Bobby became the one in four: a black male in America who'd spent some time in prison. Could have gone to Arizona.

Bobby had been locked up in a far scarier place than Bellevue, and for 200 times as many days. I'd experienced something analogous to incarceration; he'd experienced incarceration. My depression was strangling me, yet here he was, sitting with me at the kitchen table, praying for an opportunity to stock shelves, and smiling. "I'm blessed, bro, just blessed."

The world isn't obligated to help people like Bobby, but I think I am. I saw how many more hurdles than your average white suburban teenager Bobby needed to clear to earn the right to enroll in a Psych 101 seminar at Arizona, and the dire consequences of catching his toe on even one of them. And it pisses me the fuck off.

A hard-ass trial lawyer in our office once referred to us — public defenders — as "moths to a flame." We're there because we can't help it — because we can't be anywhere else. But this commitment to social justice comes at a steep price. The job attacks your empathy — the speed and ferocity of the attack varies, but everyone feels it. Like a marriage, the first part is all catalyst — a chemical reaction that can carry you through the first several years in relative bliss. It's the lull afterward that requires effort.

The older, more embittered public defenders are the equivalent of the miserable alcoholic uncle who says "Trust me, don't ever fucking get married." The honeymooners, fresh out of law school, tell themselves (and the old-timers) that they're different. They are privileged to be here, thrilled really. "We have the best job in the world," they assure one another. The statistics don't apply to them; they ignore the hard data, along with the anecdotal misery permeating the air.

If you really look at it with your eyes open, it's hard to deny that the job takes something from you. You will look older than your peers at law firms. You will not be able to afford the same moisturizers, gyms, and clothes that are the first line of defense against aging. You will become familiar with the term "loan forbearance." You will, in all likelihood, drink a great deal more than you should. All of your colleagues will reinforce on a nightly basis that this is not a problem; they will be standing next to you at the same bar, on a Monday, five whiskeys deep, pretending the suffering they've witnessed all day, week, month, year, last five years, doesn't tuck them in every night. You will smoke. Even at $13 a pack, your colleagues will always be well supplied and willing to share, no questions asked. They will know that you *need* a smoke and will often offer before any request is ever made; they enjoy saying "One of those days, huh?"

You will get angry. Here's a twenty-minute snapshot: Mr. Santos, my client, an elderly drug addict with AIDS, is escorted to a holding cell behind the courtroom. Santos is old and looks much older. He's an addict, takes methadone, and was caught with someone else's methadone bottle. That's not legal, even though there are several non-nefarious explanations for why it could have happened (e.g., maybe he was dope sick and didn't have his bottle on him). He's been in jail since he was arraigned five days earlier; this is his second appearance before the judge. The inside of his file distills his sad story into a few chicken-scratched acronyms: *AIDS, MH issues 730, Undoc Mex, Meth Px, Prog.* That's a lot of good stuff. Gives me a good *Come on* angle with the DA. "Guy has AIDS, mental health issues, has a methadone prescription. He's done a drug program in the past, gets treatment and medical attention through a program. Can't we do time served?" I leave the illegal immigration status out.

"Will he take it?"

"Imagine he will; can I have it?"

"If he'll take it today. Onetime offer."

"Fine."

"Counsel, you're up," the court officer tells me once Santos has been secured behind the bars, and I go into the back to deliver the good news through a Spanish interpreter. "You want to go home? I got you time served." Bad news: he doesn't really get it and I have five minutes, max, to make him understand what the deal is before the court officers march him in front of the judge. That's usually more than enough time to run through the magic words we have to say before the judge will accept the plea: It's a yes, no, yes, yes, yes.

Do you understand that you are pleading guilty to a crime and as a result of this plea you will have a criminal record? *Yes.*

Is anyone forcing you or coercing you to take this plea? *No.*

Have you had adequate time to speak with your lawyer about this plea? *Yes.*

If you are an undocumented immigrant, do you understand that your plea may have collateral immigration consequences? *Yes.*

Is it true that on January 12, 2010, in the County of Kings, you did knowingly possess a controlled substance, to wit, methadone without a prescription from a physician? *Yes.*

Sentence imposed. Time served.

Cuffs come off. Go in peace and sin no more.

At least that's how it *should* go. Mr. Santos's plea was routine — the judge had undoubtedly taken thirty or forty just like it by that point in the late afternoon. I'd probably stood up on six or seven of them that morning alone without a hitch. "If you get confused, don't answer. Tug on my sleeve and ask me. You understand? *Entiendes?*"

"*Sí, entiendo.*"

"What do you do if you get confused? Blank stare. You tug on me, okay? You ask me, okay? You don't answer, okay? It's okay to ask me, but don't answer any question you don't understand, okay? It's going to be yes, no, yes, yes, yes. I will tell you the answer in your ear. Understand?"

"*Sí, entiendo.*" But Mr. Santos fucks it up in front of the judge.

"Have you had enough time to speak to your lawyer?"

"No."

Shit. Technically, this is true — that he has bungled up the five magic words is irrefutable evidence of that. He'd been afforded five minutes to comprehend 500 words of legalese in a foreign language.

As soon as he says "No," I grab his arm and say, "Yes. Yes, you have."

"My lawyer?" he asks the judge.

"I'm not taking the plea!" the judge announces with some gusto.

"Judge, if you'd just…He was confused for a moment, the interpreter has translated the question again. He understands. He wants the plea. He is ready to allocute if you'll just give him—"

"Not taking the plea, Counsel. Next case. Court officers take charge." Gavel.

It's Friday afternoon, and we took too long. The judge is cranky and wants to go home; that's the real reason Mr. Santos will spend his weekend on Rikers. Five minutes of the judge's time was not worth sparing an elderly drug addict with AIDS three more days in jail. *Sorry, Mr. Santos. See you Monday and we'll try again!*

No time to wallow. I can think about whether or not I fucked that up later, because Mr. Prescott is waiting to take his own plea: fifteen days for shoplifting batteries or deodorant or whatever else he could lift from Rite Aid that has some street value. Maybe he's buying drugs with it. Maybe food. Maybe both. Either way, the folks at Rite Aid are out $35. And you, Mr. Prescott, can take the plea now and be out next week or reject it and risk them raising it to a month or forty-five days.

"I'm going home?" he asks before I can even establish whether he remembers my face or not. Santos has been swapped out with him and he's now standing in the holding cell.

"We have an offer, but unfortun—"

"Time served? I'll take time served. We can do that."

"I know you would, but that's not the offer. They're offering you fifteen. You've been locked up five days already, they automatically shave off five days for good time, so you have…five more days."

"Man, fuck that. How come they can't give me time served? Or an ACDC?"

He means an ACD: adjournment in contemplation of dismissal—it's essentially a dismissal.

"You know they aren't going to give you an ACD, man."

"Okay, time served, then."

"They won't do time served."

"Can you just ask them?"

"I did ask them. Of course I asked them. Ten times probably I asked them. What do you think I'm doing here?"

"You right. You right. Can you just ask 'em again?"

"You think they'll cave on eleven? We aren't doing better than fifteen days. That's five more days—you can do that."

"I'm not taking that shit. I'll do time served."

"Of course you would. I'd like them to kick us a little money too, but we aren't going to get that either. You want fifteen? I know you don't want it, but will you take it?"

"Ask the judge."

"I will ask the judge. Of course I will. But this judge is a dick, and I promise you he won't do it."

"Try."

"The only try I can do is say 'Will you consider ten, judge?' and he'll say 'No,' and then he'll ask if we'll take fifteen. It's a huge roll of the dice if you reject it today—next appearance they might want a month. Bite your lip, man."

"I'll take fifteen."

"Let's do it."

I am a used car salesman, but instead of cars, I am pushing bullshit plea deals. *I'll ask my manager, but I really think this is the best we can do. So what do you say, can I get you into a fully loaded fifteen-day jail sentence today?* No money down, take it or leave it.

Next, Domestic Violence Guy. It's a weak case, so the DA is willing to give me a plea to a noncriminal offense and an anger management program. So he's going home. Probably *home,* which is a problem because there is still an order of protection against him to stay away from the missus — not to call her, text her, Facebook message her, or contact her via a third party. To do so will result in new charges, but they have a kid and she wants him back and no harm will come of him going home if the cops don't find out about it — or so DV Guy and the missus think. I'll most likely see DV Guy next week or the week after on a contempt charge for violating the order. Cops will come by to check that he's not there, or more likely, the couple will have differences again and the neighbors will call the cops.

So I walk out of the courtroom with Santos, Prescott, and DV Guy on my mind — probably in that order — but happy hour is nestled somewhere between numbers one and three. *Was* Santos my fault? Could I have tried to run through the plea a few *more* times before the guards brought him out from the back? *No, not my fault. I* wasn't the one who wouldn't give the man ten minutes to understand the nuance of the guilty plea he was attempting to take. *I* wasn't the judge who just wanted to get the fuck out of there. *I* wasn't the court officer yelling at us, "Now, now! The judge is ready now! We have to move the docket along, Counselor! It's already four fifteen." Hadn't I said, "Yeah, we just need another minute. I have to explain this to my client"? I didn't have shit to do with the fact that he was a poor, sick addict. In that moment, I was the only soul left in the courtroom who ached for his predicament.

You can vent to a colleague, but that's annoying as shit. "Yes, I know. I have the same job as you. I did that fifty times this week too." Still, most of us can't help it. That's what makes the bar after work unbearable; no one can talk about anything but asshole judges, vindictive DAs who think our clients — and us too — are scum, and asshole clients who think we're conspiring against them and yell at us all day: "You work for the DA! You don't give a shit! I want a new lawyer!"

Let that shit go. Your presence alone must stand as proof enough that you care, that you are one of the good ones. Remind yourself that, pawn in the system though you may be, you are the only force pushing back against the police state, the indifference to the suffering of those who many people regard as subhuman. Let that empathy shit go. It pokes holes in you, and you *will* bleed out.

Idealistic ferocity may be impossible to sustain, but the dark secret is that morbid curiosity endures. Our profession gives us a front-row seat to our nation's most sadistic horror show. And if you think that's without appeal, I invite you to flip through your basic cable channels late on a weekend night and count how many "inside prison" reality shows are running back-to-back-to-back marathons. Whether these shows turn your stomach or not, there is an undeniable voyeuristic appeal to this barbaric institution. It's mind-bending *cruelty,* but it's mind-bending all the same. Maybe not all PDs feel it, but I'd be suspicious of anyone who denies it too forcefully.

When I was a summer intern at the San Francisco Public Defender's office, the mornings were spent trying not to fall asleep in court, but in the afternoon we'd go to San Quentin. A place where I'd be committing a crime if I brought someone a Happy Meal. Handcuffs, ankle shackles, bars clanging, guards, guns, razor wire—all that shit. Each visit was different and you never knew who or what you were going to get: could be a speed addict with face tats who'd yell at the attorney for fifteen minutes straight while the attorney yelled back, me wondering the whole time if he was going to try to murder us both; could be a baby-faced drug dealer with limited cognitive capacity who couldn't lift his eyes off the ground and clearly had *no* idea how much shit he was in; could be a stoic con who knew exactly how much shit he was in and, really, wasn't even sweating it too hard. There were infinite variations and yet they all felt utterly the same. Everyone's biography boiled down to: fucked-up enough.

*   *   *

After eight weeks of drinking and smoking in a garage in Wichita, I knew I had to go back. In some way, I missed bearing witness to the barbarity of the whole damn thing: the callousness with which an old fat white man can send a skinny black crack addict to Rikers. The judge probably doesn't give it a second thought on his way to the parking lot. He probably brags about it: "I've handed out more than a decade of jail time this week alone! I bury people under the jail." In his mind, he's a bourbon-swilling-in-chambers learned sage, not a grown man playing dress-up in a $24.99 Jostens graduation gown, banging his gavel like every order-in-the-court cliché he's seen on network TV. He probably loves it when people call him "Judge" at barbecues. I was not ready, but I couldn't stay in Wichita any longer. If only for Bobby Prince, it was time for me to participate once again in the sick joke of a justice system we've come to accept as the only logical way to deal with poverty-induced crime. To bang my head against the immovable wall of bureaucratic indifference again and have my heart broken on a loop as poor black men in cuffs were cycled through the courthouse on a conveyor belt all damn day while quietly dreaming of ripping off my boa constrictor of a necktie and running through the halls of criminal court screaming, "This is fucked! This is all fucked! This whole damn court is out of order! Attica! Attica!"

Burn it down.

CHAPTER 10

IN THE CAB FROM LaGuardia to my new apartment in Williams-burg, I remembered the familiar and uniquely New York sensation that with every second you are alive, money is rapidly draining from your pocket. Twenty minutes and $50 later, I arrived at my latest Craigslist find on the corner of Manhattan and Metropolitan Boule-vard. It looked like an old warehouse from the outside.

For the sixty days I'd hid out in Wichita, I was incapable of con-fronting the full weight and force of the fallout. Before the psych ward, I was pretty sure I was the best damn trial lawyer in the office, the next Dave Chappelle, and the coolest dude in the Village to boot.

But now that I was back in New York without the benefit of a manic episode to boost my self-esteem, I had no choice but to confront the facts. And they were bleak. A madman had raided my checking ac-count, committed malpractice on my behalf in the courtroom, and alienated anyone who had been paying attention. Didn't much matter that the madman was me. Corporate America wasn't too sympathetic to my plight: there is no overdraft protection plan that covers *I was extremely manic and purchased $800 worth of novelty T-shirts from Urban Outfitters—can you let this one slide?* You can't accuse yourself of fraud. And it's not like I had money to begin with. I made $1,400 every two weeks. My rent was $1,200 and student loans were $700 a month. An unlimited metro card ran me another hundo. By the time

I shelled out for utilities, internet, and cell phone, I was left with about $18 a day to make it through the month. It was always fingers crossed that the rent check didn't come out before my paycheck went in. Most of the planet has it worse, including anyone in need of a Legal Aid lawyer, but I did think it over before I bought ChapStick.

That first week back, I swung by my old apartment in the East Village (the one I'd covered in red Sharpie from floor to ceiling) to pick up a trash bag full of bills and delinquent student loan notices. Rather than risk a paper cut, I took a page from the Bird's pre-bankruptcy days and tossed the sack into the wire mesh can on the corner of St. Marks and Avenue A. When I was a kid, if bill collectors called the house, the Bird would hand the phone over to me to let me polish my British accent. "Don't worry, they'll call back," she'd say. A model of financial responsibility she was not, but when you ain't got it, you ain't got it. And I ain't got it. I assumed my cockney rhyming slang would get a bit of practice in the weeks ahead.

I had to reacquaint myself with adult life, but I still didn't much feel like moving. Without Granny there to cook for me, breakfast became $1 coffee from the bodega across the street. Lunch was a ham sandwich from the bodega across the street. Dinner was a frozen burrito from the bodega across the street. Dessert was my one daily indulgence, in the form of six Budweisers from the bodega across the street.

The bodega guy became my primary source of sustenance and 90 percent of my social life. Which was tough because his English wasn't great and my enthusiasm for idle chitchat was low. I don't know if he nicknamed me "Budweiser!" or if that was just his way of saying "The usual, boss?" but that was his standard greeting. My standard contribution was *Yup*. Or, if I was feeling particularly gregarious, *Yup, how's it going?* I had a few weeks left on my medical leave of absence from work, so I spent my days in bed.

It wasn't hard for me to admit I was depressed — sixteen hours of sleep nightly is conclusive on that issue—but it was hard for me to give myself permission to be depressed. Sure, I had just experienced a psychotic break that had resulted in involuntary confinement in a mental institution, lost what I believed was a real shot in comedy, lost an apartment, and lost the confidence that comes from knowing my mind wasn't going to walk out on me at any moment. But I couldn't help thinking about what Bodega Guy's life looks like when he takes his apron off after an eighteen-hour shift at Best Price Grocery. I had to assume ringing up Now & Laters hadn't been his idea of the American Dream. To him—or, really, to me when I imagined the world from his eyeballs—my life probably looked pretty decent: $1,200 for a room in a trendy Brooklyn neighborhood with a TV and a Wii. I wasn't making weekly trips to Western Union to send remittances to Islamabad, wasn't worried about my family's physical safety, wasn't worried about my legal status. Long-distance calling cards weren't a part of my life's necessities. Sleep and beer—that was the cross I bore. What right did I have?

And what about my clients? What about all the poor brothers and sisters across the city and the shit they had to deal with? Fuck, what about all the poor brothers and sisters in Syria for that matter? They sure had their hands full. What do you even call depression in a refugee camp?

Depression felt as much a luxury as veganism and fair trade coffee. *Shut the fuck up, you whiny, ungrateful bitch* constantly pinged around in my head. No matter how many doctors or Birds say it's okay to be depressed, that Wichita boy in me says *No.* He says fight. Fight through it, fight through your self-pity and your tears. Fight through the daddy-sized hole in your heart. At least you've met him. Fight through it literally if you have to. Punch someone, drink something, drink something then punch someone.

I needed a psychiatrist.

*   *   *

So I got one. Standing on the 2 train platform on my way to meet Dr. Singh, I watched a rat zipping through the puddles in between the tracks and discarded bags of Cheetos, empty Snapple bottles, old gum, and other delicious rubbish. He was a busy boy. Trying to get a few crumbs here and there, looking for Mrs. Rat, or at least Mrs. Rat Now. Dodging poison, ripping it up in the dark tunnels. Taking small delight in the terror he inflicted in the hearts of children and grown men alike. Being a rat didn't look half bad.

I've never stood on a subway platform and *not* thought about what it would be like to throw myself in front of what's coming. But I found myself standing a few inches closer to the edge, listening a little more closely to the question that the train was asking of me. I knew I wasn't going to stick my neck out on my own, but what would I do if a kid on a scooter bumped me from behind? I was pretty sure I would tighten my core and push back with the full force of my hamstrings at the first brush of contact. But I was less sure than I'd ever been. So I guess I was approaching something like *fairly* suicidal. But do you get to claim that if you'd never cut, jump, or load the gun? Feels a bit dramatic.

I made it up to Harlem and across the Columbia campus to Dr. Singh's office. I thumbed through an old *New Yorker* as I waited. Dr. Singh opened the door at 11 a.m. sharp; he looked dapper in a charcoal-gray suit, blue shirt, and purple tie. "Zachary? Come in."

I took a seat on his faux leather couch and surveyed the room: Don Quixote print on the wall, box of tissues to the left of the couch, and three shelves of scholarly tomes.

"So it's nice to meet you. Your mother called me and made an appointment — you were just in, is it Wichita, Kansas?"

"Yes."

"And you're a public defender in Brooklyn."

"Yes."

"That sounds like a stressful job."

"It can be."

"So the limited information that I have on you is that you recently had a hospitalization at Bellevue. And the preliminary impressions are that you are possibly bipolar one with perhaps a dual diagnosis of marijuana and alcohol abuse."

"That's correct."

"And the police found you on the subway with very little clothing on, you suffered a psychotic break, and for nearly a week were under the impression that you were on a TV show?"

"That is all also correct."

"Has anyone explained to you in detail what exactly bipolar one means?"

"I read the DSM-IV description and I read a little bit of *An Unquiet Mind*. I can probably describe what happened to me, but no, I don't really know what it means. Before all this, I thought it just meant you had high highs and low lows."

"It's a bit more nuanced than a *high high*." He told me bipolar disorder used to be called manic depression and then ran through the symptoms for me:

1. Inflated self-esteem or grandiosity (ranges from uncritical self-confidence to a delusional sense of expertise)

I think operating under the presumption that Larry David ain't got shit on me as a comedian suffices for this one.

2. Decreased need for sleep

Four hours max per night for an entire summer. Sometimes none.

3. Intensified speech (possible characteristics: loud, rapid, and difficult to interrupt; a focus on sounds, theatrics, and self-amusement; nonstop talking regardless of another person's participation/interest; angry tirades)

How about writing said speech on one's walls in red Sharpie when no one cared to listen any longer?

4. Rapid jumping around of ideas or the feeling that thoughts are racing

See above.

5. Distractibility (attention easily pulled away by irrelevant/unimportant things)

I spent entire Saturday afternoons filming passersby on the street. I watched a Mike Tyson documentary six times in a week because I thought I could create a blog centered around commentary of this single film.

6. Increased goal-directed activity (i.e., excessive planning and/or pursuit of a goal, whether social, work/school, or sexual) or psychomotor agitation (such as pacing, inability to sit still, pulling on skin or clothing)

Summer goals 2009: Ink deal for one-hour stand-up special. Sign contract to write in and star in TV series. Make contacts at New York Times. *Help Producer get his record label off the ground. Get my own record deal on his label. Fifty pull-ups every morning, followed by two hours of soccer.*

7. Excessive involvement in pleasurable activities that have a high-risk consequence

I think I got a bingo, Doc.

Dr. Singh is an expert on dual diagnosis—those of us who run around naked on the subway *and* like our devil juice and pot too much. He explained that some people, even those who aren't bipolar, can have psychotic episodes triggered by marijuana. Or I could be in the category of people who might not otherwise have had a manic episode but have a predisposition to those sorts of things, and pot might have been the tipping point. Or it all could have just happened anyway. No way to tell really, except not smoke and see what happens.

"But," he explained, "I am not telling you to never smoke pot again. I don't like to tell people what they can't do; I haven't found it to be very effective over the years. What I would advise, though, is that we have you abstain for a relatively short period of time—a year—and then if you experience another episode, we can know for certain that you are not one of these borderline cases, perhaps just more vulnerable to marijuana. Would you be willing to try that?"

I told him that it sounded hard, but I'd try. We talked medication and he told me he wanted me on as little as possible—that Depakote and Risperdal were heavy drugs and he thought we could probably get away with a mood stabilizer for now. *Lamictal.* Most patients have no side effects. And those who do usually get only a mild skin rash. No impotence. No hair loss. No weight gain.

For the first time in my life, I was excited to try out some psych meds. When I was diagnosed as depressed in high school it felt like a moral failing and taking pills felt weak. Yeah, I was happier on my Zoloft, and I no longer wanted to drive my car into the river, but it wasn't "real." What I was feeling now was definitely "real" and it was definitely awful. My only qualm with the new regimen was that the new meds wouldn't kick in for two or three weeks. That sounded like decades to me.

As we were wrapping up, Dr. Singh told me about the *Truman Show* delusion. There'd been some recent media attention on people who, like me, in the throes of psychosis, become convinced that they're the stars of their own reality TV shows. It's not a separate diagnosis — it's still BP1 or possibly schizophrenia. In any case, it's a rare and distinctly modern phenomenon; folks in the 1800s couldn't well imagine they were reality TV stars.

I couldn't make it through most nights without calling the Bird. By the tone of my voice, she could always tell how I was feeling before I finished my first sentence. Those beginning few weeks back in New York, we didn't directly discuss the state of my psychic health much. She just tried to pump my tire by piling on anecdotes from my child-hood. How I used to run around in my underwear and my sister's snow boots and play He-Man. How, when I was just out of diapers, I'd hold my breath until I turned blue and pound my head against the wall when I'd get mad, and she'd have to blow in my face to keep me from passing out. How she had learned to ignore the glares of strangers in the supermarket when I'd lie prostrate in the middle of the grocery store aisle, screaming and pounding my fists for an intolerably long time. How she used to have to lock herself in the bathroom and read her copy of *The Difficult Child* "so that I wouldn't have to fight the urge to beat you." How when I was five and the head of the PTA asked me what I wanted to be when I grew up, I told him, "A faggot." How I used to violently smack the ground any time I let in a goal playing soccer, and how inconsolable I'd be for hours after a loss, even at eight years old. How she "almost had to open a can of whoop ass on the parents who used to yell 'Check his birth cer-tificate!' because you were a good player and so much bigger than everyone."

Hearing these stories was comforting in a way that "You are going to be okay, I promise" never could be. "You are going to be okay" acknowledges that you are very much not okay, and the best we can muster at this point is illogical and empty assurance: you *will* be okay. Based on what? No one ever says, "You will be okay because…" followed by a compelling reason. It's strictly aspirational, patronizing even. "You will be okay" means you're in an abyss right now, and I got nothing for you. You never get step-by-step instructions for emerging from the abyss.

The Bird's stories said something entirely different. They said, "Don't lose yourself, because I still know who you are." They said, "You are weak right now, so weak that you need to hear about how marvelous I've known you to be since you were born; how unconditionally and attentively I've loved you since you got here; how I've had your back since day one, saw a truth teller where everyone else saw a little smart-ass. You were the toughest to give birth to, the toughest to raise, even tougher than your pothead brother. Yet I went to bat for you against everyone and everything, even when I should have let you face the music, because I see you, who you are, what you are. And you won't be facing this music alone either. This is just another chapter of *The Book of Zachary* I've been taking notes on and writing in my head for twenty-six years."

Of course this unwavering support took a serious toll on the Bird. As nightmarish as the psych ward was for me, what my mother had been forced to go through was probably worse. Until I regained lucidity, I had no idea that I was out to lunch. I didn't have to sit there and watch the whole thing, wondering if the guy she was so proud of was ever coming back. Things had never been easy for her: first a drunk for a father, then a cokehead for a husband, then a tyrant for a second husband. Poor the whole time, buying nothing for herself, putting every dollar and every ounce of energy into her children. Mac 'n' cheese, borrowed margarine, $3 in the gas tank. Doing it all alone with a constant headache and constant anxiety about how we'd make it.

And we kind of did: The Bird had graduated from Dillon's, put herself through college, and gotten a master's degree. And she'd kept going: at age fifty, she was closing in on a PhD in education. Alexa had gone on to veterinary school at the University of Florida, and was now in her residency at an animal hospital in Chicago. Adam was taking his time, but we knew he'd figure it out. The Bird was so proud at my law school graduation and immediately took to writing "Esq." on my mail even after I told her to quit since it didn't impress anyone in an office full of Esquires. That one of us would get pegged with the Uncle Eddie bullet had been her worst fear as a parent. She started researching signs of childhood mental illness when I was two, but despite all the shit I got into growing up—the fifteen fights, the two expulsions, the suspensions, the totaled cars, the bouts of depression—by God, her boy'd made it.

And then one day she got a phone call that her B.B.H.B.B.B.I.F. was locked in Bellevue and possibly schizophrenic, just like her crazy-ass dead brother.

The guilt I felt about the burden I was placing on her, after a lifetime spent swallowing tough pills forced on her by the failings of those around her, burned my insides. I had always dreamed about being the source of her salvation, and here I was, dragging her backward. And yet she knew and I knew, no matter how dark it got, she would be there. Ain't no quit in the Bird.

CHAPTER 11

AND THEN BLACK SANTA DIED.

The Bird was sobbing so hard I couldn't understand her. I had to tell her three times to breathe before I could make out "Terry!" and "Gorilla."

"What?" But just as she knew when I said "Edward" on the day he died, I knew what "Terry!" meant. There's hysterical crying, and then there's the love of my life just died crying. This was the latter. "When, what happened? Breathe."

"He's dead, Gorilla. He's dead. His sister found him. He was in his boxer shorts on the bathroom floor! He's dead, Gorilla!"

"When?"

"I was at school. His sister called me and asked if I was sitting down. I thought his parents died. Never in a million years did I think…Terry! Oh my God! Oh Jesus!" She sounded like she was hyperventilating.

"Bird, sit down. You gotta breathe. Sit down and breathe. Don't say anything for five breaths." I could still hear her sobbing and gasping for air, but slowly her breathing grew steadier.

"I'll come home."

"But you're not okay!"

"But *you're* not okay, Bird. I'm coming home."

The Bird looked a mess when I arrived at 1050 Denmark two days later. She told me she'd been taking Valium and that her friend Lisa was monitoring her. "I can't even remember what I done took."

"Well, by God," I said, "you're a pill popper is what you are."

"I'm a, by God, twice-divorced widow is what I am." She laughed, then cried. Then pointed to the shellacked piece of petrified wood with the lantern and the sticker of Jesus. "Fake husband gave me a piece of wood with my savior on it."

"Not even going to give you shit about your magic savior. I'm sorry, Bird."

"Old drunk. Old smoking drunk, leaving me here like a widow and a crying fool. Doctor tells him not to smoke and what does the old fool do? Dies in his underwear on me."

I'd never seen my mom so helpless. Maybe if she told herself enough times that Terry was a "fake husband" and a fool of a drunk, she could start to believe it. But the Bird is no liar. She knew what Terry meant to her. "I'm not even a real widow. He's going to have two ex-wives at the funeral and I'm not even number three."

"That's a piece of paper."

"Hombre. Oh my God, Hombre." Hombre was Terry. I don't know if the name was from his bodybuilding days in Spain or something nasty that I didn't want to know about. I chose to believe the former.

The Bird joked on the way to the funeral. Enough that I decided I could make fun of her and possibly it would make her feel better. "By God, widow at fifty is what you is."

"I can pick 'em," she said.

I was less ruthless than usual, though. Normally when she talked about Terry I'd launch into a five-minute soliloquy on his Christmas gifts. In addition to the Bird's petrified wood Jesus, he'd once given my sister a pamphlet extolling the virtues of olive leaf extract. It had clearly been inside the packaging of some sort of snake oil supplement. Terry just had the pamphlet. Alexa regifted it to me the next year. That same year, he gave Adam, a twenty-three-year-old, a wind-up NASA rocket toy and me two books I could have read in fourth grade. The Bird was furious, but if petrified wood Jesus wasn't a deal breaker, neither were these.

When we got to the church, she couldn't front any longer. I could barely hold her up as we made our way in. Julius, Terry's father, who was probably ninety but looked sixty, motioned for the Bird to come sit by him, resolving the widow issue in her favor. This pleased her. "Getting the, by God, widow's pew at least."

"At least the important stuff's going your way," I said. "We'll try to get you walking on your own accord again soon."

"No one needs your forked-tongue sarcasm in the house of the Lord."

The Bird and I made our way over to Terry's father and she buried her head in his shoulder. It had to be hard to see him — he looked a great deal like Terry would have if he'd lived another twenty-five years.

"I'm sorry, baby," Julius said. "I'm so sorry."

She wailed throughout the service. Louder than the real widows, louder than everyone.

I dragged her to the casket for that little morbid ritual. If I hadn't been capable of supporting her entire body weight, she'd have tipped over the casket. "Bird, you can't get in there with him," I said.

"But I want to. Oh my God, Hombre."

The final hymn lasted about seventeen minutes. "Jesus, oh Jesus," etc. I whispered in the Bird's ear, "How long is this goddamn song?"

She dug her nails into my hand and said, "You are in a house of God, you cynical little smart-ass."

Terry was buried in the same cemetery as Uncle Eddie. On the drive over, the Bird alternated between flippant sarcasm and grave pronouncements. "At least I got my widow status. Did you see how Julius swatted all those other biddies away? Only Terry's drunkard son had anything to do with those ho bags."

"Why do they have to be ho bags?" I asked her.

"Because *I* am the widow."

"I wonder who's calling you a ho bag in the cars behind us right now."

"By God, all of 'em can call me a ho bag because Julius knows I am Hombre's widow."

"Maybe we'll get you a placard. Attach it to some shellacked petrified wood."

"Gorilla. Goddamn. Let your mother grieve."

"I'm going to be sore tomorrow from dragging you around the church and keeping you from jumping into the casket. I'm allowing you a proper grieving."

"Hombre was never going to get a PhD like he said. I knew he was full of bull. But..." She was ready for another breakdown. "I want to play gin rummy with him. And listen to gospel music. And touch his beard. His beard. Oh my God."

"Breathe, Bird. Breathe."

"I feel like there is a swarm of bees in my armpits and a Volkswagen on my chest. And my head is throbbing."

There was comfort food at the reception: black-eyed peas, ribs, greens, fried chicken, and sweet tea. The Bird told me to go eat so I didn't become a low-blood-sugar gorilla, said she could stand on her own feet for a minute and she'd sit if she needed to. I loaded up a plate big enough to feed us both in case I could get her to nibble a little. "I bet you won't eat fried chicken, but will you have two bites of mac and cheese?" I asked her. "It's not very good. But you need your strength, woman."

"This is far more painful than my brother's death. It eclipses my two divorces. The only time I've ever felt worse than this is seeing you in the hospital."

"You don't have to rank 'em, Bird."

She ate a little and then told me that we needed to go. "If one more bitch or sonofabitch tells me I should be grateful for the time I had with him I might just whoop somebody's ass."

I only stayed a few days. I wished I could take her back to New York with me. If Wichita was responsible for so much scar tissue on my psyche, what did the Bird's soul look like? My dad, then Clyde, then her brother, now Hombre. And according to her, losing the love of her life wasn't the worst part of her year. I told her I wished I could stay with her and take care of her, and that I would if she wanted me to.

"Gorilla, you and I been through the fire with gasoline-soaked drawers on. And we're still standing. Now get your hairy ass back to New York and stay out of my garage."

CHAPTER 12

WHAT DO YOU WEAR the first day back to work after a ninety-day leave of absence due to experiencing a psychotic break? The dress code at the office was lax—T-shirt and jeans was my norm—but I churched up for day one with a sober navy sweater and pair of dark slacks. My hair had grown out and was styled, for once, in a court-appropriate fashion. Even though I knew I wouldn't have anything to do, I got there early—I didn't want to walk in during rush hour. I felt about as self-conscious as an elephant in a small law office when I pushed open the double doors of our main ninth-floor entrance. Darryl was sitting behind the reception desk.

"Hey, D."

"Uh-oh! Z. McD in the building! You back, man?"

"Back."

"All right, Zack. I see you. My man Zack back in this."

"Good to see you, D. Gotta check in."

"Check in, Zack. That man Zack checking in."

I buzzed my security card and entered the interior office. Instinctively, I walked to my mailbox to pick up my case printouts, subpoenas, and discovery material from the DA's office. Of course there was nothing there, but it was gratifying to see that my name was still on my slot. The drinking fountain next to the mailboxes was still fucked-up and patched together with duct tape. The soundtrack in the lobby was the same: "I need to speak to a fucking lawyer! I need my god-damn Legal Aid!" Darryl chilling out whoever was going off on him. Darryl gets yelled at a lot.

On the other side of the door, in the offices, a low ambient grumble of lawyers complaining about clients and DAs, punctuated occasion-ally by some of the more volatile attorneys shouting at their clients on the phone. "Mr. Green, it's two fucking days of community service! Two! And they will dismiss your case! These are criminal charges!" I took a deep breath and decided there was no use delaying it any longer: I had to go talk to my supervisor.

Just before I rounded the corner, putting myself in my boss's direct sight line, I made a U-turn back to the lobby and dove into the restroom; 213 — same code, thank God. *This is a huge fucking mistake.* I fished my phone out of my pocket, scrolled to the *B*s, and tapped BIRD. It was 8:30 a.m. in Kansas — she'd be busy setting up her stu-dents as they trickled in. She answered on the first ring; her phone had become an appendage since I moved back to New York.

"Gorilla report?"

"Gorilla at Legal Aid."

"First day of school? Not good?"

"Not good." I spilled it — sobbed, breathed, sobbed. "I shouldn't be here. This is so ridiculous. I feel like such a fucking idiot. Fucking id-iot. I can't see these people again yet."

"Steppers keep on stepping. You're a..."

"Not a stepper! Not a stepper. No steps."

"You're a leaper, Gorilla. Three months ago you were in a goddamn psych ward. You're at work now. You're still an attorney. It's not easy, what you're doing."

"I want to leave."

"You can leave. Can't you?"

"Technically, I guess I could."

"So if you want to leave..."

"Of course I *want* to leave, but this is stupid, right? I shouldn't be scared of these people, right?"

"Who scares you? What are you scared of?"

"Everyone. And everything—all the time. The subway. Confined spaces. Walking through the halls, waiting for everyone to stare at me. Madman back in the building."

"You need Mama Gorilla to open up five cans of whoop ass on somebody?"

I knew she'd love to. "You know what? Fuck this. Fuck 'em all. I'm doing this."

"Puff out that big gorilla chest and go rip it off like a Band-Aid. Call me if you need me."

I wiped my eyes, left the stall, and splashed some cold water on my face. *Don't let them see you sweat. Steppers keep on stepping.* I looked in the mirror—*You look good, you look normal. You're a normal guy.* Then I slapped myself in the face as hard as I could. Game time.

I swiped my security card again. Round two. I passed by the paralegals' bullpen and gave a friendly wave to Chele and Jana. Both stood up and smiled, but I kept charging—figured I'd act like I belonged here. My supervisor's office was steps away and I saw him before he saw me.

"Barry." I hit him with a two-fingered salute.

"Mr. McDermott! Look what the cat dragged in. To what do we owe the pleasure? Are you *back* back?"

"Yeah, I think I am," I said.

"Well-hell-hell, we are thrilled to have you."

"Good. I'm thrilled to have you as well, Barry."

"And there he is," he answered. My sarcasm seemed to relax him. "So I guess let me call the powers that be and see what the procedure is. Do you have a note? I think they'll need a note."

"Shit. I had a note"—I did have a note—"but I forgot my note." I left out the part about being too busy trying not to throw up as I forced myself out the door to remember the note.

"Okay, I'll call Dawn and see what the deal is. There's an open office where Jenny used to sit. I'm not sure if you're still going to be in our cluster, but if you are, it will probably be in there."

"Okay."

"Good to see you. Stand by and I'll get in touch with Dawn."

"Ten-four, boss."

I felt emboldened after my talk with Barry. He seemed genuinely glad to see me. More important, he didn't seem to look at me differently at all. I sat in my new temporary office, a downgrade from my first office. There, if I craned my neck, I could *just* see the Statue of Liberty behind me. Now if I craned my neck I could *just* see three beige walls and a giant beige filing cabinet, all bathed in white fluorescent. After half an hour or so, Barry came into my office looking a bit somber. "So I talked to Dawn. You need a note."

"Okay," I said.

"You actually can't be here without a note. Sooo...you're going to have to leave until we get one from your doctor."

"Can I have him fax one? I could call him right now. If I reach him, I imagine he could shoot one over right away."

"Sorry, you can't be in the building."

"Okay, no problem."

"It's just a procedural thing."

"Them's the rules," I said, trying to show that I knew they weren't *his* rules.

Relief and dejection washed over me as I bundled up: I was able to leave, but I was also not allowed to stay. For all the lip service people in my office pay to the notion that mental illness is no different than cancer or diabetes, I couldn't help but think that Teresa from the immigration unit wouldn't have been sent packing after returning from chemo if she'd forgotten her note. Would they even have asked her for a note or would her new short hair and the fact that she was standing upright be proof enough that she was fit for duty? The note rule didn't feel like the fulfillment of a bureaucratic requirement; it felt like a request for proof of sanity. *We're thrilled to have you. Now we'll be needing certification that you're no longer certifiable.*

By now the entire office was trickling in and milling about in the halls. Obvious double takes were quickly followed by polite smiles and trailing "Welcome backs." I was on display, and I could tell that some of them hadn't expected me to return. As I made my way toward the exit, I quit making eye contact with people. *Pretend you're just leaving to grab lunch, like it's any other day.* Who was I kidding? I was just going to waltz in here in a cardigan and suddenly everyone was going to forget that I'm crazy? PDs are, for the most part, a nonjudgmental bunch, but we ain't above some good ol' fashioned office gossip, and I figured I knew what today's topic would be: *Did you hear he's back? I wonder if they'll let him go to court. Is he stable? They sent him home.*

Toward the end of my first week back, Barry came 'round to fetch me for the come-to-Jesus talk I knew was coming. He was borderline sheepish as he informed me that I'd been "away" when they'd done performance evaluations. I wasn't sure if he was referring to my geographic location, my state of mind, or both. From there, we proceeded to a completely nonconfrontational stare down. I assumed he was thinking *Come on—do I really have to say anything?* That's pretty much where I was at too: sympathetic that he actually had to address my indiscretions in measured, middle-management speak. I thought about his possible lead-ins: *So, uh, don't strip at happy hour, please—we all got wind of that one. Show up to work, please, preferably not two hours late every day. Please consider how you'd feel if you were a seventy-one-year-old first-time criminal defendant and your twenty-six-year-old attorney came to court in a fucking Mohawk. Oh, and don't email me to ask if you can use my Yankees tickets after you've been AWOL for two weeks.*

Barry's approach was soberer. Like any good dressing down, he started with some compliments. "You have the potential to be a great trial lawyer. You're good on your feet. You read people well, you have good instincts on cross, and you're charismatic. But—and this is one of those scenarios in which everything before the 'but' doesn't carry much weight—you are underprepared, you mail it in, your files are a mess, your voicemail box was full and had been for months. You're late every day. You wrote one motion all year. It was good, but it was one motion. It's great that you tried a case and it's great that you won. But, honestly, it was an easy case. You had no idea what you were doing, you had a great judge, and you nailed the guy once when it mattered. This is not a knockout punch business, though. We win by working the body. Look through the transcript. You probably missed ten objections that would have been a big deal in an important case."

All true.

I had a solid insanity defense and a sympathetic jury, but I wasn't going to try to defend "my" conduct. Barry knew what happened. He's a Legal Aid lifer. For more than thirty-five years, he'd made his butter begging for mercy for tens of thousands of people who'd done bad things they wouldn't have otherwise done but for drugs, poverty, and mental illness. Barry understood that sometimes there's a Bellevue pit stop on life's itinerary.

I pled to the docket—guilty on all counts—and tried to own it. I told Barry that I knew I'd let everyone down. That I was embarrassed. That I knew I was lucky to have a job and to work with folks who understand a DSM-IV code. That I'd been sick. Really sick. And that I was better now.

"Listen," he said, "this isn't Skadden, Arps, LLP, or some other white-shoe fart factory. This is Legal Aid. We're all a little bit nuts. If we're not when we get here, we are by the time we leave. Nearly everyone here has some big trauma in their past life. We're underdogs. That's why we do it."

"True."

"Welcome back. I'm done playing supervisor now. They make me do it a few times a year."

It didn't soon get easier to walk through the Legal Aid lobby every day. In order to reestablish myself, I was playing a character every bit as much as in the Myles days. Zachary Myles McDermott, Esq., said things like "Boy, I feel like it's just about latte time. Am I wrong? Did you catch *Breaking Bad* last night?" He laughed when people answered the latte proposition with something like "More like beer o'clock," even though he knew Debbie wasn't *really* up for grabbing a beer at 3 p.m. He listened when people told their stories about rote interactions with judges and DAs; he clucked at their generic tales of injustice and laughed at oft-recited lawyer jokes. He did favors for people when asked and he told people in kind "You're a lifesaver. You're the best!" He even once said "Cold enough out there for you?"

That was my next six months. Since my caseload had dropped from eighty-five to zero, I was mostly pulling "catch" duty, covering cases for colleagues who couldn't make it to court—a shit system for everyone involved. It was par for the course not to say a word to a client before we were standing next to each other at the podium. Within sixty seconds, I was handing the thoroughly confused defendant a yellow slip of paper with his next court date scribbled on it while he was told, at a volume well beyond reasonable, to "Step out of the well!" by the court officer. I wanted to do more: go into the hall and explain to every client the ins and outs of Fourth Amendment search-and-seizure jurisprudence and its implications on the constitutionality of modern stop-and-frisk. But, fuck, I had eighty of my colleagues' files to get through and people mostly just wanted to know if their case was going to get called or if they should just plan to die in the courtroom. So it was easier to keep the international *One minute* index finger up at all times and look through people like they were wind as they stared directly at me and shouted "Lawyer! Mr. Lawyer. Mr. Lawyer!"

That or sit in my office waiting for the world to make more internet. I had to laugh at myself, thinking I was going to come back with piss and vinegar and start shoveling sea stars back into the ocean. Excessive enthusiasm was about as useful as adrenaline coursing through a DMV clerk's veins.

After a day's work, I'd go home and fall asleep almost as soon as I stepped through the door. It helped that it was February and the sun started setting not too long after lunch, but 5:30 p.m. is still a bit early to shut it down for the day. When I'd wake up every few hours, I'd squeeze my eyes closed until I fell asleep again. Life couldn't touch me when I was unconscious.

I tried to tell myself that the Lamictal would kick in and boost my serotonin levels in due time, that it would change things, just as Zoloft had in high school, when I shifted from depressed Zack who would sit in his car and cry to Grammy Award–winning Christian rock band Creed to the Zack who did his homework and ran wind sprints on his own after practice. Where was that dude? He had to be in there somewhere, but he felt like a distant friend from childhood whose last name I couldn't remember.

As people sometimes do in lonely times, I began to think I needed a girlfriend. I came to believe that my German ex-roommate and I had been in love. I also came to believe that if I could just get her in a room, I'd be able to talk her into being in love with me. I texted her and kept texting her: Just a breakfast? Nothing. I just want to talk. Nothing. I won't try anything. Nothing. Such a cold German heart. Nothing. You don't miss me a little bit? Nothing.

Then, sitting in my apartment, seven beers deep, it came to me: Must talk to you now. Emergency. Herpes.

And I got a reply: That's fucked-up. What the fuck are you even hoping to accomplish?

I thought I'd been clear on that point: Just a breakfast?

We never got breakfast.

I was fucking bored. And I knew if my Bobby Prince–generated potential energy didn't swing toward kinetic soon I'd end up like the crusty old drunkard PDs—coat on at 4:58, eyeing the clock until 4:59, out the door at 5:00 with a fifth of vodka in my briefcase, ripping Newports until my teeth turned into popcorn kernels. It's a job where you *can* coast, and this shit is dull as church if you don't apply yourself.

I went home at the end of every day with tight shoulders, in a shit mood but unable to attribute it to one thing in particular. It was always a variation of the same fight with the same opponent; the blows were familiar, hard and steady from all angles. Was it the mass incarceration that had me down? Was it the judge who told an intellectually disabled grown man with forty-three misdemeanor convictions that since he didn't learn the last time with a thirty-day sentence, let's see if sixty would teach him a lesson? Was it the private lawyer in orthopedic shoes, half-untucked shirt, chili-stained tie, and pit-stained suit jacket who told his client in the pen, "I'm not Legal Aid, okay? I'm private," like he was Johnnie L. Cochran Jr. himself, raised from the dead. The same guy who then, for reasons unknown, yelled at his client, "That's why white women won't sleep with you. Because you're an asshole thug." The misery just bleeds together. You feel sorry for your clients, but pity is adjacent to contempt. Constant conflict and suffering rests in the back of your psyche, even if you *had a good day at work.*

But occasionally there's a client you remember and feel you can do something for—something beyond the mere call of professional duty. I pulled up Case Tracking—our janky 1987 MS-DOS database, and typed "Miller Jr., Earl" in the client field. I expected his case to be closed—dismissed and sealed 730. Actually, I wouldn't have been shocked if he'd picked up a few new cases in the four months since I'd last seen him, corrections officers dragging him by his ankles back into the pen. *Fuck outta here!* But his case was still open. New attorney of record: Alinari, K. How could his case still be open? The mentally incompetent standard is tough to establish, but Earl thought threatening to burn his building down was nothing more than a landlord–tenant issue.

I knocked on Alinari's door. "You get a case of mine?"

"I got twenty cases of yours, McD."

"Did you get a crazy guy, charged w—"

"I got nineteen crazy guys charged with something. Go on."

"Earl," I said.

"Miller Jr.," she said.

"Yeah, what's up with that case? I thought I 730'd him," I said.

"You did."

"Fit? He's fit?"

"*Found* fit. But he's definitely *not* fit," she said, and I knew what she meant.

"Is he still on Rikers?"

"Yup."

"Fucking serious?"

"Fucking serious," she said. "He came back fit. Earl Jr. has been trying to cop a plea for several months, but Judge Arriaga wouldn't even allow him inside the courtroom on his last appearance. I get him all set to take the plea—he's got the time in by the way, just needs to plead guilty and then he can leave—and we've tried four separate times to allocute. He's fine in the cell one minute, then he's screaming at me calling me a stupid bitch and talking about burning the place down."

"Can we do anything? Can you re-730? Advance his case?" I liked the way the words sounded in my mouth—it felt good to get the lawyer slang back.

"I don't know if you can *re-730*—never tried that before. That's a question for Special Litigation if you feel like walking upstairs," she said. "He's on again in three days, though, so probably no faster way of getting him out than trying to get him to stay calm for five minutes and plead guilty."

I asked Alinari if she wanted me to come to court with her, though I wasn't sure it was the best idea in the world for Earl to see a "familiar" face. I doubted he'd recognize me, but if he did, it might get the persecution wheels spinning in his head.

"I'm taking Drinkwater. He's the plea whisperer," Alinari said. "If he can't get him out, we'll figure out what Special Lit can do. Don't sweat it. It's not a big deal. Let's get lunch this week. I have a Rikers call in ten with my twenty-seven-year-old mandatory persistent felon. Two-victim shooting with witnesses and a confession. They're offering him twenty to life."

"Good luck."

Twenty to life. That's the shit that really terrified me about being a public defender: quarter-century stakes. I didn't want to be the goalie in front of that net. I almost threw up the first time I saw a young man get cuffed in the courtroom. He came into court as an "INVOL"—involuntary return on a warrant—meaning he'd missed his court date and the warrant squad picked him up and hauled him in front of the judge. He'd been arrested for jumping over the turnstile. Usually, the judge will just give the INVOL a new court date or another chance to do community service. But on that day, maybe because there were new attorneys watching from the front row of his courtroom, Judge Wilson threw him in. Fifteen days in jail for failure to complete a few days of community service—scrubbing subway cars that had been filthy beyond redemption for decades. No one was in the audience for the boy as the court officers slapped the cuffs on him and led him to the cell. The DA called him a "transit recidivist," said he'd done it three times before, meaning the city of New York was out $2.00 x 4 turnstile hops = $8.00. That's how it came to pass that an old white judge with an old white beard ordered a young black man to be led away in chains, crying and begging for mercy as two thick-necked officers smiled and dragged him away. I was certain it wouldn't be the last time he saw the inside of a Brooklyn jail cell. I doubted he'd ever graduate from high school or eat an organic chicken breast with roasted chickpeas and kale. Eight bucks: *Get in the cage, boy.*

At four months and counting, Earl was serving the longest sentence of anyone I'd represented up to that point. I wondered if his fate would have been different if someone other than me had picked up his case at arraignments. Maybe some other newbie would have written a brilliant motion to get him out. But I had peaced out to the hospital where Earl belonged. Now he was stuck in New York's largest mental health facility: Rikers Island. He thought he was going home when he met me. *Fuck outta here,* he was sure of it. Men in riot gear now patrolled his housing unit with mini fire extinguishers of pepper spray attached at the hip. Rats crawled on him while he slept. Other inmates probably took advantage of him; aside from being crazy, Earl also seemed to have an intellectual disability. Did the guards take him out of view of the cameras and beat him when he flew off the handle? I've had more than a handful of clients tell me that it's the corrections officers everyone is really scared of on Rikers, and mentally ill inmates are frequent targets.

I was pretty sure I'd done everything by the book on Earl's case and that it wasn't my fault he'd been on Rikers for four months. Alinari is a great attorney and she hadn't been able to get him out either. But if I was going to eventually move into the big leagues and start handling heavy felonies—the cases where we argue about decades, not days—I would have to put my incompetence on display and ask the questions I didn't want to have to ask but damn well should. Or I could stay in my lane in misdemeanor court—no balls required.

*   *   *

I'd had about enough of my sad, boring job, my sadder boring life, and my 5:30 bedtime. I missed Zack. I missed his life pre-Myles. I missed Myles's crazy ass too. Pre-Bellevue I was big-wave surfing in Maui; now I was doggy paddling in septic lake water. I took a survey of my situation and decided I had to start reconstructing some sort of human connection to supplement my late-night phone calls with the Bird.

The one piece of my pre-Bellevue life that remained was Jonas Jacobson. I first met Jonas when he gave a lecture at UVA Law—his alma mater—about pursuing a career in public defending. He started his speech by writing $145,000 on the blackboard. Everyone knew what that meant: the average starting salary for our peers in the private sector at the time. Then he erased the 1, leaving $45,000 on the board. "That's being a public defender right there," he said. "The first thing you need to ask yourself before you get into this work is 'How much of a consumer am I? How much stuff do I need?' One hundred forty-five thousand dollars is a lot of money. Think before you turn it down." Jonas did ten minutes on the three not-guilty verdicts he'd recorded in his short career—"Three-oh, undefeated. You get to hand someone their freedom! You say 'Here you go,' and they go home to their family." Of course he had long hair and a Peruvian bead bracelet on his wrist. He pinned his hair behind his ears every few seconds and he said "zealous advocacy" four times. I couldn't decide if he was exceptionally cool or a huge douche, but I heard enough to know I was a PD. When I asked him if it was possible to live in New York on $50,000, he told me, "I'm alive." We stayed in touch through the Legal Aid application process and he shepherded me into the Brooklyn office. Without question, I was a Brooklyn PD because of Jonas Jacobson.

Jonas, age thirty-one when I started at Legal Aid, slept on a twin-size mattress on the kitchen floor of an East Village apartment he shared with two of his brothers and Dr. Al. His little brother had taken over his room when he briefly moved in with his now ex-fiancée. Little bro sold pot. Big bro was an unemployed Harvard Law graduate. Dr. Al, big bro's college roommate, age thirty-six, an actual doctor and father to a sixteen-year-old, had bunk beds in his room for when his daughter stayed over. It all made very little sense, but I liked it. Jonas would often extol the virtues of the "K-room" (aka the kitchen) to anyone who would listen: "I pay no rent. If I need to piss in the middle of the night, I just stand up and pee in the sink. I have my reading lamp. I lay in there and read the *New York Times* on Sunday mornings. I own nothing. Nothing. You can fuck in the K-room. I fuck in there all the time." He sold it with such enthusiasm and sincerity that occasionally I'd find myself wondering what was so wrong with me that I hadn't yet found a K-room of my own. But then I'd remember we were talking about sleeping on a dirty three-foot-by-six-foot kitchen floor. At $0, he was paying just above fair market value.

I missed him, even though I consistently declined his invitations to hang out. He understood that I was in a dark place and didn't take it personally, but I owed him a yes. So toward the beginning of spring, when he threw a party at his place, I bucked up and went.

As soon as I got there, I realized I'd rather be home asleep. It was too loud and too many people were having too much fun. I wished I could upholster myself in black leather and become one with the couch. Up to that point, it'd been fairly easy to stay away from the reefer, but I was damn near contact high with all the smoke in the air. After an hour, my brain began to turn: Would one toke of the stuff really shoot me straight up the bean stalk? What was so good about being on the ground? Dr. Singh himself had said he wasn't so sure it was the pot that had caused my psychosis. Best to abstain, yes. But it's also best to eat food, not too much, mostly plants. After forty-five minutes of nursing a beer, when the joint came around for the fifth time, I said, "Fuck it, let me hit that."

And: nothing bad happened. I got high. I got drunk. I started telling stories about my uncle Randy, who showers with dish soap and keeps a gallon of water next to his toilet. I don't know what it's for. I owned the room for a solid five minutes, and I remembered how good it feels to hold court—to not know what you're going to say next but to feel unafraid all the same. I flirted with anyone who appeared to be unattached. I didn't get laid, but it seemed like I might again someday. I felt like a guy people might want to be friends with.

It was the first thing I'd done since Bellevue that felt just about right. Age-appropriate—albeit situationally risky—recklessness. So I kept doing it. And nothing bad kept happening. Jonas and I started going out together three times a week, barhopping, chatting to girls, and I came to appreciate the therapeutic power of getting laid semi-regularly. I never found the defrost button for depression, but I stayed alive and put the turkey in the sink and it eventually thawed out on its own. Shit got better because hard shit usually does.

Normal-ish felt incredible for a time, but that Myles guy I'd stuffed in the closet—he wasn't dead. It was impossible to snuff out a corner of my personality that had once so wholly defined me. The itch to perform, to create, was never going away, but I was scared of it. Picking up a pen or a microphone felt riskier than hitting that first joint.

But I had to try, with new rules: No losing sleep to comedy or writing, hence disregarding the comic's rule that if you think of something at 3 a.m. you must get up and write it down. And if I *did* have to write something down at 3 a.m., bullet points, not paragraphs—if it's good, it will make sense tomorrow. Weed seven times per week, no. Weed two times per week, tentative yes. But no smoking after midnight and no smoking once initial high has been achieved. Don't allow delusions of grandeur to substitute for work. It's okay to toil away in secret.

I had plenty of trepidation about going down the rabbit hole again, and I didn't know how much, if any, of my break was attributable to comedy. Could I pursue creativity at 85 percent? Was I good enough to get anywhere by giving less than 110 percent? What if I found that I needed to go a little crazy to hit my potential — could I settle for mediocrity in order to keep mentally stable or would I go all in at the first whiff of opportunity? I didn't know, but those sounded like good problems to eventually have.

I ran it by Jonas over a sushi lunch at our regular spot on Smith Street. He started gently shaking his head no. "Don't you think that kind of fucked you up?"

"Maybe. I don't know. But I have to do something. I don't even know if it's stand-up, but I want to write or hold a camera. Make a documentary. Act, even. I don't know."

"So you're just going to go buck wild again? Full-on Myles, with your Mohawk and shit?"

"No, but I think I've got to see what Zack's got."

They say write what you know, and I realized that my biggest appeal to The Producer had been that I could be at home in both the Lower East Side and a trailer park. Christmas was now just a few weeks away and I was looking forward to a voluntary trip to Wichita. Always plenty of material in the 'Ta. I talked Jonas into coming home with me. After all the hillbilly stories I'd told him about the McDermott side of the family, he didn't need much convincing. I was eager to see what these humble folk would make of my womanizing Jew buddy. Quite possibly they'd think we were lovers, especially with his moustache. I was even more excited to watch him watch them.

That afternoon, we booked tickets from JFK to ICT.

CHAPTER 13

ON A WINDY KANSAS day, you can smell Grandad's garage from the end of his long circle driveway: Scott's lawn fertilizer, potting soil, and fuel. There's always a brand-new Cadillac parked in the garage (that's his church and rent collectin' car), a Chevy three-quarter-ton with a $75,000 fishin' boat hitched to the back (fishin' truck), and a GMC work van filled with what looks like the entire power tools section of Lowe's. My dad's father made his bones in real estate; a self-made man with little respect/time/patience for anyone too lazy to ascend from rural poverty to McMillionaire status. He's in his eighties and a bit hobbled, but he still gets the van out to his rental properties in the Wichita community of Planeview, his exurban empire and a sprawling crack den of a neighborhood, six days a week: "patchin' roofs, changin' out a radiator, fixin' a winda." Grandad collects rent in his Cadillac on the first of every month, "'Cause if ya waits any longer, they spends it." On the Seventh Day, he follows the Lord's command to rest by working on his lawn and garden until it's too dark to see. He built the house Jonas and I were about to enter with his bare hands.

Christmas Eve at Grandad's goes like this: We feast on deer chili. The chili is not good—the fat coagulates and simmers at the top of the pot and the end result looks like a public school lunch from a poor district. Uncle Frank—my dad's stepbrother—is in charge of the scoopin', which means after first portions have been doled out, he walks through the dining room, pot nestled under his armpit, bellowing like a mess hall cook, "Who wants another scoopin'!?" Most of the crowd will indeed want another scoopin'. These people — my extended family — eat like they've just broken out of prison.

Before he serves the chili, Frank usually stares into the pot as if he's on an acid trip. He's more or less preserved in a state of timeless ugliness; he never looks any older from visit to visit, but not because he's aging well. His beard starts just below his eyes and ends an inch above his nipples, lending him the air of a Confederate soldier nearing the end of the war. This year, like every year, both his baseball cap and T-shirt featured a variation of a bald eagle tearing through the center of an American flag, and both were caked with oil and grease. I've seen him remove his hat so few times that I always forget he's entirely bald on top. The sides and back of his hair are long and dirty. Frank had all his teeth pulled due to general rot when he was forty-five — a birthday gift from Grandad. You can tell he stinks from twenty yards away.

I sidled up to Frank — motioning for Jonas to join me — as he continued to zone out on the final few stirs of the pot before the blessing.

"What's up, Frank?"

"Same shit."

"What have you been up to?"

"Not shit." He never redirected his gaze from the chili.

Per tradition, Frank didn't wash his hands before helping with the food prep. The grease and oil under his fingernails and filling in the cracks of his weathered hands could be yesterday's or last week's.

At least one-fifth of my extended family in attendance at Grandad's house have done crank at some point. Frank for sure.

Jer'my — as Grandad pronounces it — is Frank's son and also a member of the meth contingent. He was dressed like a rodeo clown in a bright red, pearl-snapped Wrangler shirt tucked into painted-on Wrangler jeans tucked into red boots. A Colt .45 was holstered on his right hip, and two sheathed knives were attached to the left side of his belt. When I said hello to him, his response took the form of a question: "Guess how many beers I done drank today?"

"Um, twelve?"

"Sixteen. And half a pint of whiskey." Beaming with pride, he didn't slur, even slightly, as he let me in on this little secret.

"Do you have a lipper in?" I asked, knowing full well the answer.

"Yup, Cope. Black. You wan' one?" he politely offered.

"I can't, but thanks. Could never handle Copenhagen."

"More for me."

Jer'my tried to hide the fact that he was dipping by swallowing the brown juices, but the faded ring permanently branded into the back of his jeans revealed that he partook regularly.

Cousin Tater was also there after a five-year boycott on account of his sister marrying an Asian. I applauded him on his journey; he even expressed a desire to have his Confederate flag tattoo removed from his shoulder. Said the Lord told him to.

Uncle Randy practically ran to greet me when he looked up from the Walmart shrimp cocktail he was shoveling into his mouth by the fistful. Instead of a normal hello, he made the international "OK" sign with his thumb and forefinger and placed it on his belt. "Hey, man, you know what that is?" He did not wait for me to answer before launching into his explanation. "In high school, we used to play this game, man. If your friend walked up to you and went like that, you had to poke your finger through the hole—otherwise it meant you was a faggot."

"That makes sense," I said. "If you don't penetrate your male friend's hand pussy, you're probably gay."

"Please, white boy. I used to get more ass than a toilet seat. Where's that girlfriend of yours, that blondie?"

I didn't know if he meant my high school or law school girlfriend. Both had been subjected to several of his unsolicited hugs.

"I don't know where she is. I don't have a girlfriend right now."

"She was sweet, boy. She was sweet on me."

"Probably. Toilet seat and all."

"Hey man, I got a bone in the van if you want to sneak out later."

"We might could do that." I slip into Wichita vernacular quickly when I'm home. It's a hobby. If tradition held, in a few hours, Uncle Randy would be in the garage challenging me to a push-up contest on our knuckles, followed by a stomach-punching contest. He'll struggle to snap off more than three or four push-ups — his gut is sizeable — but the frozen December concrete will irritate his knuckles not a lick. Once the punching contest begins, I'll remember why: his knuckles are made out of frozen December concrete, hard as they are sharp. I always forget that he punches like a wrecking ball until he knocks the wind out of my solar plexus and then strikes the exact same spot with his second punch, doubling me over. "See, that's how your granddaddy taught me to punch, way back, boy. This before your time." He'll continue his tutorial until he hack-laughs himself into a coughing fit. Odds are decent that he'll moon me too and tell me to "tell all them Yankees that they can kiss my Rebel ass!" followed by another hacking, coughing fit.

"Aw'right!" Grandad shouted. "Get in here! We're gonna say the prayer, then we're gonna start the scoopin'!"

It's the same prayer verbatim every year. His voice lowers from rootin' tootin' Arkansas sharecropper to somber televangelical preacher.

"Lord, we thank thee for these blessings you have bestowed upon us. We thank thee for these gifts, and we ask thee to bless this food that we might use it to nourish our bodies so that we may glorify thee. You loved us so much that you sent your only Son down from heaven. Jesus, you loved us so that you died on the cross for our sins. In your Son's name we pray. Amen. Let's eat!"

"Oh, man. Let's get this chili, boy! Who's scoopin'?!" Uncle Randy was so excited to eat the chili that he jumped on a chair and assumed a position that was half chicken flapping its wings, half man shitting in the woods. "Oh, man," he whooped, "I been ready for this for weeks. I didn't eat all day."

The rush to the pot had all the urgency of a Black Friday door buster at Walmart. Despite the fact that there would be leftover chili for days, and that he would certainly take seconds and thirds, Uncle Randy filled his red plastic Solo bowl beyond capacity until chili ran down the sides and onto his fingers. He licked the chili off his hands and proceeded to pile half a pack of Dillon's-brand shredded cheddar cheese and two handfuls of stale oyster crackers on top. The bowl was buckling.

After dinner, we all went down to the basement to open presents. There are hunting lodges with fewer animal heads on the walls and rivers stocked with fewer fish than Grandad has displayed in his basement. Ten-point buck, elk, catfish, and stripers. No saltwater fish. Their fake, sad marble eyes look down upon us and ask *Why?*

Adjacent to the elk wall is a gun cabinet that houses a small arsenal. The first time I saw a gun fired was in this basement. I was eight. Grandad, sixty-five at the time, somehow spotted a snake near his pond from at least seventy yards out. "Get down!" he boomed as he ran to the gun cabinet. He was locked and loaded within seconds. I dove behind the couch and lay on my stomach like a G.I. Joe. *Boom!* "Got 'em!" He had not bothered to step out of his house before firing the gun through the open basement door; as he discharged his weapon, he rested his leg on his Barcalounger.

The gift exchange on Christmas Eve is actually more of a small redistribution of wealth. Despite Grandad's disdain for welfare recipients — "See, first you get one black, and then she's sixteen and she gets pregnant. Now you got two. And then, see, she gets pregnant again. And now you got three. And they's all on welfare, and who's paying for it? You and me. You and me" — Grandad still revels in the spectacle. Before the cash is handed out, he always starts with a joke. As he's gotten along in years, they've become more long-winded and nonsensical. The punch line is usually something along the lines of "The old man didn't report his wallet stolen because the thief was spending less money than his wife."

Not to be outdone, Uncle Randy responded with a joke of his own: "Why did Obama quit giving speeches?"

Oh boy. I held my breath.

"Because every time he got up on his soapbox, they sold him down the river!" Randy was all grins.

Next, the high point for most of the attendees: the cash. Grandad stands center stage in the basement as an ever-expanding group of sugar-high great-grandchildren scream and swirl around the carpet like little white-trash tornadoes. There are new additions every year and I've long since given up trying to learn their names.

"Jer'my!"

Jer'my snapped to attention and met Grandad at the center of the room, where he'd collect the same envelope we'd all been receiving for the past twenty-five years: Merry Christmas from Bank of America — a wreath and a bow on the outside of the envelope, Ben Franklin's face peeking through the oval slot under the flap, "Love, Grandad and Grandma." Jer'my promptly emptied the festive envelope and tossed it into the trash pile in the middle of the floor — $100 into his wallet quicker than a drug transaction.

My cousin Stacy had been staring at Jonas all evening. He's a good-looking guy — blue eyes, thick dark curly hair, strong jawline, short but extremely fit. Like her siblings, Stacy attended a Bible college in Missouri (or Mizz'er'a, as my relatives pronounce it). I'd be surprised if she'd ever had a beer or been past second base. But despite evangelical prohibitions against experiencing sexual desire outside the confines of marriage, she was absolutely lusting after Jonas. So she flirted with him through fellowship — conversation in the service of glorifying Jesus. "No offense," she said, "but why aren't you with your own family?"

"Oh, because I'm Jewish."

"Sorry, but you don't look Jewish."

"Thank you. I'm glad, because Jews are some ugly motherfuckers. Big nose, big ears."

"Yeah," she answered matter-of-factly. The notion that he even *might* be speaking sarcastically did not register.

Once all the hundreds had been handed out, Uncle Randy demanded everyone's attention. "Hey, everybody, listen up! I got a gift. I got a gift fer Dad. I want y'all to see this." Then out of his back pocket came an unwrapped rusty blade. The handle was made of a deer foot — hoof, fur, and all. He knelt down on one knee and presented it to his father as if he were bestowing Excalibur upon him. The room went silent for a moment, then...universal awe and jealousy. "That's a nice knife, Randy!" "Whar'd you git that knife?" "That's a nice knife!" "Dang, that's a nice knife!"

I can't say I was entirely unimpressed, but Grandad appeared to be. *Goddammit, Randy. That knife won't cut shit*, his face said. *I have raised a failure — three failures.* Randy; my dad, Mack; and their sister, 'Lou 'Lou. ('Lou 'Lou used to drive a school bus and is hands down the most successful of his three offspring. Her husband, Donald, is also her stepbrother. The only thing husband-stepbrother Donald said all night was "Get me one a 'em," in reference to a piece of pecan pie.)

I was actually a bit surprised at how unimpressed Grandad seemed. This was a far more appropriate gift than I'd ever expect from Uncle Randy. Grandad likes knives. Grandad likes to kill deer. Grandad likes to preserve artifacts from the killing of deer. What's not to like?

If you ask Grandad how Randy is doing, he'll say, "He's waiting for me to die so he can get my money. They all are." He's not wrong. Grandad is a slumlord and his net worth is probably in the neighborhood of half a million. That's certainly a small fortune in Wichita — enough to keep him in a new Cadillac DeVille every two years and a new work van and fishin' truck every other year. "I figure why not buy it. I can afford it. Everyone else is just going to fight over it when I die. They all want this house, but none of 'em can even pay the taxes on it. Randy is a bum. I've built an empire, and I got no one to hand it off to."

"Okay, we got one more thang," Grandad shouted, high on the adrenaline of lording his wealth over his impoverished family. "You know every year we do a gag gift, s'what I like to call it. So the boys is gonna get a tool. It's a flashlight you can put on your head for when you's fixing a car. And the girls is gonna get a smell-good candle. It's a boys' pile and a girls' pile. Everyone gets one."

Uncle Randy opened the plastic packaging with a knife and immediately strapped on his headlamp and shined it in my eyes. He was wearing a leather biker vest over a dirty tie-dyed, vaguely Native American–themed T-shirt. He was also sporting a leather top hat with a metal skull-and-crossbones pendant affixed to the middle. The look was more magician than Harley-Davidson owner. "That's real snakeskin around the brim," Uncle Randy bragged when I mentioned I liked the hat. "You can't get these here. This is down South stuff. Speaking of that" — we had not been speaking of that — "I ever tell you about the time I jammed with James Brown?"

"You've played with James Brown?"

"Shit, yeah."

"Like the Godfather of Soul James Brown?" Jonas inquired. "Hardest-working man in show business James Brown?"

"There's a lot of after-hours stuff you don't know about, man. Most of the good stuff comes out after the shows, when the musicians have their private sessions."

"You were privy to the inner-circle jams?"

"I played with a lot of guys, man. James Brown, Muddy Waters, B. B. King—he used to come around all the time—Ray Charles just once, Lynyrd Skynyrd." The Skynyrd claim was the most believable; he could at least pass for one of their roadies.

"I got a new album coming out." Uncle Randy has had an album "coming out" since I was old enough to understand what that meant. "I actually need to talk to you about that. I could use some connections out your way."

"New York?"

"Yeah, I've got some contacts there. We went through the Bronx at night once when we was out there. That's something you don't *never* want to do."

"Yeah, I guess not. You've played a show in New York?"

"We was passing through. On a tour."

This was assuredly 100 percent bullshit, but I couldn't be certain whether he knew it was bullshit too.

"Yeah, well, let me know whenever you get out there," I said.

"I will, man. I'm getting my money together. This one, I'm telling you, this one is going to put me on the map."

"Cool."

"A lot of stuff happens on tour," Uncle Randy continued. "I ever tell you what we did to my buddy passed out drunk?"

"No. What'd you do?"

"We greased up his butthole and stuck goose feathers in his ass. He woke up and didn't have no idea what happened."

"No, I don't suppose he would."

"Like I said, a lot of that stuff happens on the road."

I fixated on his teeth and, for a moment, marveled at the incongruity of his dental hygiene vis-à-vis his general bodily hygiene. Then I remembered that it had been a package deal when Frank had his teeth pulled. Grandad had decided it was only fair to extend the same offer to Randy—and so, several years before their fiftieth birthdays, both men had all their teeth extracted and were outfitted with dentures. I was certain that neither had felt any shame in this, and also that Randy would gladly remove his teeth and show me his gums if only I'd ask.

From the chili feed to the presents to the conversations that followed, I filmed everything. Jonas acknowledged that the white-trash factor was more than he ever could have possibly anticipated.

Uncle Randy declared he was heading out, but not before making a big show of hugging Grandad and telling him, "Dad, I love you." Grandad looked more annoyed than touched. "Okay," he said. His face said, *You love my money, you lazy fucking idiot, and that's all you're getting for the rest of the year.*

Jer'my offered to take Jonas and me on a gun tour. In addition to the gun case in the basement living room, there are yet more in the back utility room, which also houses the remains of Grandad's elaborate train set.

"How many guns do you own?" I asked him.

"Legal or illegal?" he answered proudly.

"Both."

"Well, I got six shotguns plus three sawed-offs, two Glocks, two pistols, a .45, and I'm getting a semiautomatic. I sleep with the sawed-off and the Glock."

"Are they loaded?"

"Shit yeah! An unloaded gun is a worthless gun. What are you gonna do if a nigger comes in your house and tries to rob you? Ask him to hold on a second while you load your gun? I don't think so."

"That's a fair point," I said. It was clear that Jer'my wanted *nothing* more than the opportunity to shoot an intruder in his home. I fully expect to learn someday that he has accidentally shot a friend or family member.

"You wanna go spotlightin' when we get outta here?" Jer'my asked. I'd never hung out with Jer'my before, but I was intrigued.

"I have no clue what spotlightin' is," I said.

"It's when you drive around in a field until you catch a deer with your headlights and you get out and shoot it. It's easy."

"Uh…is it illegal?"

"Shit yeah, it's illegal. But they just take your license away and it's a thousand-dollar fine."

"That's not too bad."

"And if we don't get a deer, we can just shoot a cow."

"I imagine that's more illegal."

"Yeah, and the farmer sometimes tries to shoot at you."

I *did* want to go illegal hunting with Jer'my. I'd never shot anything in my life, nor did I have any desire to, but I wanted to bear witness.

"Can we film it?"

"Shit yeah, we can film it. I got some Jack in the truck too."

"Done."

I gave Grandad a hug and began the arduous process of making my escape. I'm Grandad's favorite merely by virtue of the fact that I'm a lawyer in New York and, thus, I "make a lot of money"—or at least so he thinks. He asks "You at six figures yet?" every time he sees me.

"Not quite," I say, but I wink at him to suggest that I just might be.

"Hey, me neither," he always answers, enjoying our little conspiracy. Two self-made men engaging in a secret language that none of the rest of the family can understand. "When you leaving?"

"Soon. Couple days."

"You gonna come out to the house again before you take off?"

"I'm going to try to."

"Come out and eat a baloney sandwich, will you?"

Baloney sandwich is Grandad's preferred lunch. Two slices of baloney and one slice of cheese with Miracle Whip on white bread, washed down with a thermos full of coffee and a Coke.

* * *

While I didn't want the senseless death of a doe on my conscience, I reasoned that Jer'my had killed hundreds of deer in his lifetime and would surely kill hundreds more. Someone had to document this, and Jonas seemed up for it. One thing about my family is that they are not shy in front of a camera; maybe that's not a shock in this age of reality TV, but most of them have the attention-whore gene. I pointed my iPhone at Jer'my and asked what we were hunting for.

"Deer, cow, niggers, chiggers, and spics—anything that moves."

"Yup, that'll work," I answered, excited to interview him further. "Let me ask you a question, Jeremy."

"Shoot."

"You ever try any hard drugs?" I wanted to know about meth.

"Nah, nothing too hard. Just coke and weed and occasionally if I ain't got no coke, and I'm on the road, I'll do a little meth."

"Yeah, so nothing too serious."

"My dad used to do meth back when he was truckin'. He don't run truck no more, but that's why he ain't got no teeth."

"That is actually shocking to me. I can't imagine Frank doing meth."

"Well, he done it. That's why he ain't got no teeth."

"Are you scared of losing your teeth?"

"No. I don't give a fuck."

"Right."

We drove around for a few hours while I continued to grill Jer'my about his sex life, drugs, alcohol, rodeo'n, the blacks, shooting shit, and electronic communication. Here's what I learned: "A Houdini is when you's doing a girl doggy and you spit tobacc'a juice on her pooper and put it in her ass. I done that and she was none too pleased." "I like coke and meth but Jack is better." "Rodeo'n gets you tons of pussy." "Niggers steal." "Shootin' shit is the shit." "I don't fuck around with the internet or email or any of that bullshit."

"Really, no YouTube?"

"I seen it, but I don't fuck around with it."

I could have listened to this shit with interest for a long time. I am amazed by Jer'my and alternately amazed that Jer'my does not amaze me — so foreign yet so familiar. But like binging on a few hours of trash TV, there's a point when you must turn it off. I hadn't been drinking much of the Jack, but I still had to drive clear across town, and I was definitely buzzed. I told Jer'my it was about time we turned in for the night. "You sure you don't wanna get us a cow 'fore we do that?"

"I think I'm good on a cow," Jonas said.

"Well, I'm a shoot something at least. Pull over and I'll shoot this Jack."

"Of course."

Jer'my stepped out of the car and took an enormous pull from the bottle and walked it thirty or so yards down the road. He took a final swig, emptied it, and set it on the ground. Standing a few yards away from the passenger side, he took aim and fired. *Click*. No gunshot, just *click*. "This fucking thing's jammed!"

"Well, okay then."

"Nah, fuck that. I'ma shoot this fucker." He cocked the shotgun again and fired, but to no effect.

"All right, dude. Let's call it. Sorry."

"Fuck that." He ran over to the bottle of Jack and lifted the *loaded* shotgun over his head with both hands in the motion of a lumberjack chopping wood. "I'ma smash this motherfucker!"

"Jer'my is that thing…" *Smack*. The bottle didn't break.

I imagined Jer'my squinting down the barrel of his gun like a cartoon character before getting his head blown off. "Jer'my! Loaded gun!" *Smack*. Thank God, the shotgun-axe shattered the bottle without discharging.

"Fucking piece o' shit," he said as he got back into the car. "I'da been fucking pissed off if we'd a seen a fucking deer."

We drove Jer'my back to his truck at Grandad's and shook hands. "How can I get in touch with you, being as you don't have a phone and all?" I asked, half intending to actually follow up.

"Just call Grandad. He knows how to get in touch with me."

He spit a huge wad of Cope on the ground and fired up his truck. It was the loudest gunshot of the night.

CHAPTER 14

GETTING TRASHED ON CHRISTMAS has been a tradition in Wichita since high school. Before hitting the bars, Jonas and I secured some pot from one of my high school friends and went to see *True Grit*.

Jonas didn't know it, but I hadn't slept much the two nights prior. High off the Christmas Eve chili feed and spotlightin' with Jer'my, I wrote for hours after he'd gone to bed. I didn't want to forget one racial slur or one goose feather in Uncle Randy's friend's butt. I typed page after page of dialogue, notes, and scenes. It all felt too *good*. I knew I was flying too close to the sun. But that's the problem with feeling good—nobody ever says "I feel really good. No, like really, really good. I need to stop feeling this good—time to change something here."

It came on fast and furious, and in the moment, manic judgment won out. *I can handle this,* I thought. I was like an addict being seduced: *Just one hit won't hurt me.* Sleepy and dreamy and euphoric, dangerous thoughts turned to reckless actions disguised as epiphanies: *Ride the wave. This isn't full-on mania. You're still able to recognize it; surf on. If you have to have this disease, at least benefit from the gift part.*

I started going through old stand-up notes.

-I bet Michael Stipe cries on purpose a fair amount.
-Why is back hair so reviled? You have some chest hair—sexy.

Beard — sexy. Back — dear God, get that stuff away from me. And it's not like one doesn't foreshadow the other.

-What would the Wright brothers say to Maverick from *Top Gun* if they met?

I'd always liked that Wright brothers joke but I'd never been able to get it to work onstage. I kept thinking I should go to bed, but there was a little voice in the back of my head saying, *You can do whatever you want. You don't have to explain yourself to anyone.* I almost felt enlightened as I let that little mantra reverberate.

After *True Grit*, we hit the Burger King drive-thru. Borderline manic, I was still beaming from the masterpiece I'd just seen as we placed our orders. I tried to get Jonas to agree with me that it was quite possibly the greatest movie of all time, or at least there was an argument to be made that it was the best Coen brothers film.

"It was good, wasn't great." He was entirely uninterested in pursuing this topic.

"You're right, it's probably still *No Country,* but that movie was the shit." He didn't even answer me this time. I started to feel self-conscious: Was I making any goddamn sense? Or was my friend just a simple bastard? He probably couldn't name five Coen brothers films, I decided.

"Are there going to be any girls out tonight?"

"Absolutely. Everyone in the 'Ta gets hammered tonight."

We hit Larry Buds — a sports bar, like almost every bar in Wichita. Jonas rolled a tight little joint in the parking lot. It hit me quick and hard. "This shit is really fucking strong, don't you think?"

Jonas was again unimpressed. "You really think this is as strong as some purple haze back home? You out of your mind? This is some 'Ta weed."

"Yeah, I hear you, but I feel stoned as fuck. You aren't high?"

"I mean, not that high. I can feel it a little."

"I'm fucking stoned. Let's go inside. Save the rest of that."

It felt like half the eyes in the bar were on us as we entered wearing skinny jeans and V-necks. The women's faces said, *You don't see that every day.* The guys' faces said, *Look at these faggots.* I warned Jonas to be careful; in New York, if you unknowingly hit on someone's girlfriend, it's not unheard of to make friends with the guy once he returns. *Hey, I was just hitting on your girlfriend, sorry. What's your name?* No one takes umbrage. But in the 'Ta, you better make damn certain a girl is by herself or be ready to throw down if you're wrong. Sometimes it doesn't even matter if any of the guys she's with is not her boyfriend. I've been threatened for hitting on "my sister," "my friend's little sister," and "my friend's ex-girlfriend from high school." Also, people pack heat in the 'Ta. Many bars have a NO FIREARMS sign in the window, which always reminds me: *Holy shit, you are allowed to have firearms here! By default!*

Pitchers and beer towers of Bud Light flanked by giant plates of nachos covered most of the tables. Men yelled about the Chiefs or the Royals or the Wildcats or Wichita State or Kansas basketball—fans of each school accusing the other's supporters of being gay. I'd never left Wichita for an entire calendar year without visiting, and I spent the first eighteen years of my life here. But as the years away added up, my visits started to feel like anthropological undertakings.

It was the little things: Bass Pro Shop hats with fishhooks clipped to the brim, cutoff Kansas State football T-shirts in the middle of winter, knives on belts, camo on anything, Skoal spit into beer bottles. The only black people in the place were being piped through the sound system, save maybe one preppy black guy who had definitely been told since high school "Not you, Aaron—you're basically white."

The bar area was packed—"assholes to elbows," someone pointed out. Everyone was bumping shoulders and jostling for position. I tried to take up the least amount of space possible by turning my torso perpendicular to the bar and using my shoulder to hold my place in line. My attempt to shrink had the opposite of the desired effect.

"Hey, that's a nice beard you got there," the cowboy next to me said.

"Thanks." What was I going to say— *You making fun a ma beard, son? We gotta problem?*

"Lemme ask you a question…" Muscle memory was kicking in and I had to remind myself to dial down my inner smart-ass. *Keep the Wichita inside. Don't get in a fight.*

"That yer hand touching my leg?"

"Well, my hand is in my pocket, and I am rather squished in here, but if part of my hand brushed against you through my pocket, I apologize and assure you that it was unintentional. How about I move over here just a couple of inches? Then I won't bump into you again. Does that work?"

"That should work. I just ain't no faggot."

"No, of course. Nor am I."

"It's just you got all that chest hair showing. And that beard."

"Are the homosexuals fond of beards these days?"

"It's pretty queer."

"Okay, good to know. Nice to meet you, sir." It took me twenty-five years to learn that the last word isn't worth much; it's okay to let your adversary leave satisfied that he got the best of you. That way, you can avoid having Crown Royal bottles smashed over your head and your teeth kicked in by three separate pairs of boots. Between the two, I've found the Crown Royal bottle to be less painful, but brass knuckles trump all. I've never won a fight.

When I found Jonas, he was talking to a circle of girlfriends, frequently mentioning that he lived in New York, and oblivious to the table of men mad-dogging him directly to his left. Even if the local yokels weren't *with* these women, they still might see fit to protect them. It's impossible to exaggerate the prevalence of "He-bothering-you-ma'am?" heroism among this crowd.

Meanwhile, I'd been spotted.

"Crack McPerm. Look at you, motherfucker."

Searfoorce.

"Take a shot with me."

We tossed back something awful that no one should be drinking after their college years, probably a Fireball. Searfoorce was a high school buddy, the varsity soccer captain our senior year.

"How's New York?"

"It's good. It's really cool."

"How much is your rent?"

"Twelve hundred dollars for a shoebox with two roommates."

"See, that's retarded. I have a *house,* and I pay five hundred dollars: two-car garage, finished basement, three bedrooms, a yard."

"That would be cool. I just don't really want to live in Wichita right now." I added the "right now" because halfway through my sentence I worried I might sound condescending.

"I see you're already wearing skinny jeans. Can your nuts breathe in those things?"

I told him my nuts were okay.

"It's just gay."

I held my tongue, eyeing his baggy Abercrombie jeans with the bottoms dragging on the floor, his short-sleeved T-shirt over long-sleeved T-shirt, and his backward KU hat. Back in high school there wasn't much separating us. We took the same AP classes, got similar grades, went to the same parties, recited the same *SNL* skits, dated the same girls. But in college, Searfoorce never eased off the throttle when it came to drinking and he slowly flamed out. Eventually, he told his parents he'd graduated — and even participated in the graduation ceremony — despite being six credits short.

"Anyway dude, it's good to see you, Crack McPerm," he said. "I heard you're doing stand-up in New York. That's fucking awesome. That's like, my dream life."

"Yeah, it's awesome," I lied. I had no desire to clue him in on what had so abruptly halted my little experiment, doubly so since his eyes were already bright red and watery. At every high school party, you could set your watch to Searfoorce puking in his hands. He'd shake 'em dry and keep going. Seemed like it was getting to be about that time.

"Dude, you should come back to my house after this and watch the Northwest soccer highlight reel. I watched it the other day. We should've beat Saint Thomas, dude. For real. We could've won State."

"Yeah, maybe."

Jonas and I went out Irish, leaving Searfoorce to puke or find someone willing to break down tape on the 2001 Saint Thomas Aquinas game.

Jonas and I had been driving for nearly an hour when he realized something was wrong. I'd had more to drink than him, so he agreed to drive. "Did it take this long to get to the bar?" he asked. "Seems like no."

"It didn't."

"Are you lost? In Wichita?"

"I know where we are, but I can't really figure out the route home."

"Doesn't that mean we're lost?"

"I know where we are; just let me think a minute. Take a left at the QuikTrip."

Jonas let out a deep breath and flicked the turn signal aggressively. I could tell he was both annoyed and suspicious that I wasn't being completely straight with him.

"I feel like we've passed that gas station five times now. Are you sure you're all right? You were acting weird at the movie, but I thought you were just feeling it too hard."

I was *still* feeling it too hard. *True Grit* was banging around in my head; it had been too funny, too perfect. I wanted to watch the entire movie again and type out every line of dialogue. I felt I was unique in my ability to catch and appreciate every nuance the Coen brothers had injected into the film. Replaying the dialogue felt like recalling an epic live performance of your favorite song by your favorite band. Even if the entire audience is rocking out, you're convinced you appreciate the details — the bass line, the snare, the riffs, the lyrics, whatever — on a different level. Copying the movie seemed almost imperative. I needed to put Jonas to bed and pull my laptop out. *Hypergraphia: condition characterized by an overwhelming compulsion to write. But* can't you *feel* manic without *being* manic?

When we got to the light, I changed my directions and told him to go left. He didn't move when the light turned green. "You just said take a right. I've been driving with you for three days here and you've never once even had to look at your phone for directions. Now we're driving in fucking circles. Are you okay?"

"No." Straightforward and honest enough, but not much help to a New Yorker lost in Kansas. "I know where we are. I just can't tell you properly. You have to do the exact opposite of what I'm telling you."

"What?"

"My instincts are exactly wrong every time I tell you to go left or right. So if I tell you to go left, you should go right. Then we'll be going the right way."

"Dude, do you know where we're going?"

"Well, no, but I know how to get us there."

"Do you realize you're making absolutely no sense?"

"I know it might *seem* like that, but think about what I'm telling you. I've been wrong one hundred percent of the time, so if you do the opposite of what I'm telling you, you'll be doing the right thing. Two negatives equal a positive, you know?"

I did recognize all the landmarks we were passing, but each time we arrived at an intersection, it was like I'd been struck with directional dyslexia. My thoughts were cycling so quickly I couldn't hold one in my head for more than a second. My double-negative plan had initially made so much sense to me, but then I realized that if I kept changing my mind, I'd mix correct and incorrect instructions. Fuck. A negative times a positive equals a negative, and for my plan to work, I needed to be able to hold the incorrect answer in my head long enough to relay it to Jonas so that he could do the opposite. I decide to fake the funk: *Don't think, just react on instinct. You are in your native habitat.*

Three turns later I'd navigated us out of the Wichita city limits and into the sticks. We were barreling down a dusty country road with barren cornfields on either side of us. Jonas slammed on the brakes and put the car in park. "Are you okay?!"

"No."

"Are you fucking around?"

"No."

"Do you need to go to the hospital?"

"Yes."

"Do you want me to call the police?"

"Yes."

Jonas stared at me. "Are you sure you want me to call the po?" We were still public defenders, after all, and seeking help from law enforcement wasn't exactly second nature to either of us.

"No..." My voice started to tremble, and then I exploded, "But you have to do the opposite of what I say, so you have to call them!" I jumped out of the car and started sprinting down the dirt road. I was desperate to be understood, and mid-sprint, a genius plan came to mind. *What does Jonas know about my first episode? That I was found half naked on the subway. I have to reenact it to the best of my ability!* I started stripping as I ran. I untied my boots and tossed them to the side of the road; my shirt followed, then my pants. I was flying. It was eighteen degrees outside and the field was frosted over. If this didn't convince him that I needed to go to the hospital, I didn't know what would. I was also trying to get us back on track: If he wouldn't listen to my directions, maybe I could run him back to the highway. He'd have to follow me or I'd freeze to death.

Jonas floored it down the dirt road and slammed on the brakes a few yards ahead of me. I started banging on the window, begging him to let me back in, but he wouldn't. Maybe he was scared; maybe he was just biding his time, assessing proper protocol for a situation like this, whatever it might be.

Finally he unlocked the door, but he got out of the car as soon as I got in — ostensibly to retrieve my clothes, but he seemed more concerned with creating a buffer between us. Once he'd gathered up my boots, shirt, and pants, he drove us back onto the highway. He would have called 911 immediately, but what could he tell them, "I'm on the corner of cornfield and cornfield"?

Things escalated on our journey to find a government agency that could help. Along the way, I asked Jonas if he wanted me to stick my fingers up my ass. He declined. "You can put your fucking clothes on if you want, though." Instead I reclined the seat of my grandma's '88 Corolla station wagon, turned over on my stomach, and proceeded to get a couple of fingers in there.

"This is going to be such a laugh tomorrow, though, isn't it?" I asked him.

"No." His answer was sharp, borderline rude. "Hey, though, do put your clothes on."

I hit my head against the passenger side window and told him, "Just throw me out of the car!"

He said he'd never do that.

"Don't let me jump out of the car!"

"Dude," he said, "don't jump out of the car. You're not going to jump out of the car."

"Just throw me out of the car!"

"I would never do that."

I was worried I would or wouldn't be tossed out of the car. Every fifteen seconds, the desirable option seemed to switch. Then I'd start breathing again and try to convince Jonas that it was all going to be a big laugh tomorrow.

"No, it's not," he kept saying.

Prude.

Jonas eventually found a firehouse. He pulled up and ran inside. I knew my brain was going haywire, but I still had a loose grip on reality. I was relieved to be there; I knew I was where I needed to be. Manicked, panicked, and fucked but still marginally lucid. When Jonas came back outside, he said to me, "Don't say anything about the weed."

"No shit, I got this now."

Upon the arrival of the EMTs, I explained my condition to them — told them I was bipolar, I'd been hospitalized before, and I was having a manic episode. They asked me if I would get into the ambulance. I said I would. They strapped me down.

CHAPTER 15

THERE WAS NO MEDICAL equipment in the room, only two chairs and a TV. The attendant explained nothing, told me to take a seat, flicked on the TV, and walked out of the room.

A doctor with thick dark hair and a thick dark beard appeared on the screen; he could have been me in twenty years. "Hi, Zachary." It scared the shit out of me.

"Are you talking to me?"

"Yes, you're Zachary, right?"

"Yes."

"And you live in New York?"

"Yes."

"And how old are you?"

"Twenty-seven."

"And why are you here?"

"I'm bipolar, I'm having a manic episode, but no psychosis, and I'm not a danger to myself or others." I knew it was important to work those magic words into my file.

"Have you ever been hospitalized before?"

"Yes. Look, you know all of this shit already. I know what you're doing and I don't like it."

The screen seemed to be flashing back and forth between images of the doctor and images of me — his face, my face, his face, my face. Then the images appeared to be morphing into each other — my eyes, my upper lip, his hair and cheeks, my mouth, then the inverse. *Why are they doing this? Are they trying to see if I'll notice that they're manipulating the images?* It seemed like a cruel way to test a possibly psychotic person's perception of reality. "What the fuck is going on with the TV?"

"What's going on with the TV, Zachary?"

"It's changing. It's changing from me to you. I can see it changing. It's both of our faces. My face, then your face, then both of them mixed up."

"I'm not sure what you're talking about."

"Yes, you are. You know exactly what you're doing."

"What are we doing?"

"Just stop it! I can see what you're doing with the feed. You can stop now. It's pissing me off."

"Stop what?"

I cut him off by getting up and leaving the room. I had no idea whether I'd just passed the test or failed miserably — or if I was even being tested. *Am I going psychotic again?* I knew enough to know that I wasn't in a typical waiting room; if I stayed, I'd be locked up, but if I could hold it together and make a move right now, it was possible I could still walk out of here.

The receptionist was reading an *Us Weekly* while a junkie yammered on about needing some cigarettes right fucking now.

"What the hell was that?" I asked the receptionist.

"What was what?"

"That video shit. What was that?"

"What do you mean?"

"Why were the doctors messing with the feed?"

"Messing with the feed?"

"This is all a trick, huh? I know what's going on. I need to sleep."

"They are trying to find you a bed, I think."

"What if I just write on a sheet of paper that I am an attorney and I am not a danger to myself or others and I do not consent to being here?"

"Are you sure you want to do that, sweetie?"

I wasn't sure. But my instinct was telling me to get out of there. Bail, before it's too late. "I don't want to stay here. I want outpatient. I want my Granny. Call my Granny. I want to go to her house. She'll pick me up." I was still connected enough to reality to know that the Bird was visiting Alexa in Chicago and wouldn't be coming to get me.

"We can call her, honey, but are you sure you don't want to be here?"

"I don't know. What do you think I should do?"

"That's up to you. What do you think you need to do?"

It sounded like a riddle. Does saying I *want* to leave mean that I'm not *fit* to leave if any rational person could tell that I needed to be there?

"I want to leave."

Granny was at the psych ER in twenty minutes. She smelled like my childhood. But she had her funeral face on—I hadn't seen her like this since Uncle Eddie died. I swallowed the Risperdal the nurse gave me and we stepped outside. There was ice on the ground and I was so tired I needed my eighty-year-old grandma to prop me up. Granny is a stout old farm girl and she managed to lug me into the car. I was starving, ready for her to cook me some bacon and eggs at 4 a.m. I figured she'd be more than happy to.

"We need to call my mom," I said as I sat down at the breakfast bar back at her house.

"It's really early, son."

"I need to talk to her."

Full of unbridled manic joy from having managed to talk myself out of an involuntary stay at the psych ward, I called the Bird.

"Hey, boy," she groggily answered.

"Bird! I've figured it out. I know what I'm going to do!"

"What are you going to do?"

"I'm going to get Uncle Eddie's old chain wallet. I'm going to take it back to New York with me and I'm going to wear it! But first Granny is going to fill it with cash! I'm going to leave Wichita with a pocket full of cash! Granny is going to give me a few grand! I know she is."

"You don't sound too good, Gorilla."

"Mom! You're not listening to me! I have a plan. I want that wallet and I want it full of cash!"

"Where are you?"

"I'm at Granny's. She's cooking me bacon and eggs."

"It's four in the morning. What are you doing at Granny's?"

"I just told you."

My grandpa was now up and reflexively placed his own order of bacon and eggs. Granny served us both, then sat on a stool at the bar and stared at me. She started to cry, hard.

"Granny, why are you crying?" I asked as I put my hand over the phone.

"Son, what are you talking about?" Granny asked.

"I want that wallet, Granny. And I need cash. I need cash. Granny, look at me. Do you have any idea how quick I can flip ten grand into a hundred? Six months."

"Let me talk to Mom," she said. I handed her the phone.

"Cin-Cin, he's not good," Granny sobbed. "I just picked him up at the hospital. They said he was running through a field. He's not good... Cin-Cin, I can't handle him. He's out of control. He's so muscular, just like Uncle Eddie. But he was so weak I practically had to carry him to the car..."

She hung up the phone and told me that the Bird was going to call Dr. Singh.

"That's a great idea, Granny. He'll make you feel better. He'll tell you I'm okay."

I finished my breakfast and stretched out on the couch in the TV room. Instinctively, I punched in 32 — ESPN. *SportsCenter* was on, but I suddenly became unbearably agitated and it was impossible to sit still. I decided I needed a blanket pallet, like Granny used to make for me when I stayed home sick from school. "Granny, come make me a pallet." She did. "Granny, rub my back." She struggled to lower herself to the floor and began rubbing my back, no mention of how odd my request was.

Manic as all hell but clinging to lucidity, I knew I needed sleep and I thought the back rub might do the trick. But she just couldn't get the pressure right—first too hard, seconds later too soft. My temperature felt like it was rapidly fluctuating. One moment I was freezing, the next I was uncomfortably hot. "Just stop!" I snapped after a few minutes. "You're doing it wrong." My grandpa stood in the doorway of the TV room, breathing heavily.

An hour passed before my mom was able to get ahold of Dr. Singh and call back. When the phone rang, I was army-crawling into Pa's bedroom closet, so restless that I *had* to move but unable to stand up. The scent of the carpet, Pa's old pool cue from Ki'rea, the coffee can full of commemorative quarters that he used to save for me—everything was exactly where it needed to be and it overwhelmed me. I was time-traveling back to my rug-rat days and simultaneously warping into the future—to a time when these coins would be dumped into a sorting machine at a local branch of Intrust Bank and when the coffee cans would be recycled and the ties and shirts bagged and dumped into a Salvation Army bin. And I could feel the birthday parties of my childhood and the heaviness of the rolls of quarters he'd hand me and the Sunday dinners, when he'd still be in his short-sleeve button-down and old brown tie before changing into his blue Dickies jumpsuit for dinner. I could even feel the games of pool at the USO hall in some South Korean city. I could feel his whole life stretching out on a continuum and I could feel, sure as shooting, his death. I started to cry.

"Son, please get up. We're taking you back."

CHAPTER 16

Bird's Journal (12/27/10)

Z back in psych ward. Ran through cornfield naked. Granny picked up from psych ER. Z cackling on phone. Booked 911 flight back from Chicago.

By the time Granny and Pa were able to load me into the station wagon, I thought Pa—dressed in his signature blue Dickies jumpsuit—was actually Jonas wearing an old man mask. His breathing was labored; he was exaggerating the part to play it convincingly. I immediately rolled down all the windows in the car and froze my grandparents out. After a few minutes, I rolled them back up and blasted the heat. This continued all the way to the hospital. I was perplexed as to how Jonas-disguised-as-Pa knew his way around as he navigated the icy roads. Maybe he had an earpiece and someone was giving him directions?

Psych ER (12/27/10)

Z kicked partition in transport van from ER to Good Shepherd psych ward—van took him back to psych ER. GS decided to send him to state hospital—they won't take violent patients. Van to Osawatomie State Hospital scheduled to pick

Z up at 9 a.m. tomorrow. Called Dr. Singh — he told doctors no history of violence. Re-admit to GS.

When I woke up the next morning, it didn't even occur to me to question why I was eating breakfast in a cafeteria full of strangers. I picked up a bread roll and threw it at another patient's head. Luckily, it missed. There was no ill intent; I think I just thought it was funny — like starting a middle school food fight.

My second psychotic break was ignited and burning white-hot — a wildfire of madness feeding on itself, torching every corner of my brain.

After breakfast, we were escorted like a group of preschoolers to the ward's main corridor. There was an alcove on the left side of the hall with a recliner and a TV. I walked down the hall, surveying the people and my surroundings. When I got to the end, I pivoted and began to run wind sprints down the ward's corridor, dodging the zombies along the way. I had Olympic speed; maybe it had always been there and I was just now learning to tap into it. The orderlies told me to stop sprinting, but I couldn't. I ran the length of the hall two or three times and then pretended like I was going to quit so they'd leave me alone. But it felt too incredible to be that fast; I was flying and I couldn't stop. The staff overlooked it for the time being.

Later in the morning I was called into a room where five or six doctors and nurses sat around a conference table in a semicircle. I offered to take off my clothes and drew some things on a dry-erase board. Then I started to chant in a vaguely Gregorian style, only I pushed the air out of my lungs as violently as possible, the result sounding more like an elephant seal in heat. "Sorry if that smells like halitosis," I said. "I haven't brushed my teeth in eighteen hours." One of the doctors snickered. The rest stared at me with *What have we here?* expressions. *They are in awe of me,* I thought.

And then I broke it all down for them:

"The best way for me to explain my mind to you is like this: Think of yourself as a robot. Think of all the functions your body is performing simultaneously and successfully. Think how incredible it is that you are even able to stand upright and walk with an even gait, that at the same time, your eyes are taking in and processing thousands of stimuli and your brain is attaching a label to every single one: puddle, crack, dog, woman, bald man, car, shitty car, asshole in a suit, mother, father, doctor. Think about how remarkable it is that you can walk by a brick wall and estimate within a margin of 10 that there are probably about 540 bricks in 18 rows of 30—you count, you're off by 8, not bad. Is it wrong to conclude that, maybe, you are superhuman? After all, who else can do that? Who's to say you aren't plugged into the universe a little bit deeper than everyone else? That you can almost *see* the subatomic particles and energy fields encircling the pretty brunette walking down the street. 'Look at me,' your mind commands. She does. If that ain't power…

"Now, most people can probably tap into this on a certain level—you are more plugged in than a homeless guy, for example. So why can't I be on a higher mental plane than you, in the same way that you're above the homeless guy? Where you see two steps ahead, I see six.

"But here's the kicker: That homeless guy on the bench muttering to himself—the one with the dreads and the army surplus coat that looks like it's been dragged through a filthy gutter then rubbed in shit—he feels this shit more than you do. It's the main reason he's homeless—he's consumed by it. I know because I stop to talk to these people. *These* guys are on my level, and you dismiss them outright. Before the internet existed, someone had to babble some crazy shit about a connected interweb of computers talking to each other. Explain it to an alien; you can't. It makes no sense. Neither did cells at some point in history, but now we can see them. You really don't think we'll ever be able to see atomic molecules the same way? Can I go? That's all I've got for now."

One of the male doctors told me to go back to the common room. I understood. I had blown their minds and now they needed to discuss.

By the end of my second afternoon at the Good Shepherd psych ward, I was convinced that *I* was the Good Shepherd himself, possessing the power to heal the sick—a useful skill in a hospital. I felt the inner peace and fearlessness that Jesus described: *Be not afraid, I go before you always.* I'd heard it a thousand times before, but now I *felt* it. I approached a patient in a wheelchair and began to blow on his foot in order to restore his power to walk. He laughed so hard tears poured down his face. *Ye of little faith.* I knew he'd experience the miracle soon enough. Jesus must have walked around feeling pretty smug with all of those miracles stashed in his back pocket.

My first round of wind sprints was frowned upon and I was chastised. The second round landed me in seclusion—an eight-by-eight-foot room with padded walls and a tiny square window. I immediately panicked and began to bawl uncontrollably. Pounding on the door, I pled for mercy. "Please let me out! I'll be good! I'm sorry!" The orderly on the other side of the glass ignored me. "I'm suffocating in here!" This was a cruel solution to a problem I couldn't understand.

Gasping for air, I lay down on the padded floor and tried to breathe. It wasn't easy, but eventually I began to realize that the only way out of this box was to demonstrate that I was calm. After a minute or two on the floor I tried again. Tears streaming down my face, I simply looked at the attendant, hoping to silently unearth some mercy. His indifference was unflappable. "Look, I'm calm now. Look at me! How long are you going to fucking keep me in here?! Look at me!" I yelled.

He wouldn't.

Back to the mat, I decided that I must meditate. I breathed in deeply and exhaled fully. *Take twenty breaths. Take twenty breaths.* I assumed a Muslim prayer position — folding at the knees, tucking my legs behind me, and reaching forward to the wall — and summoned the help of all the deities I don't believe in. My knees ached — arthritis from my soccer days — so I flipped back over and lay in Savasana. *Breathe.* I placed my toes against the wall and pushed. The wall moved. The wall moved! *If Jesus could move mountains with the faith of a mustard seed, why couldn't I push a wall an inch or two with my toes?* An intense calm washed over me and I felt equipped to manipulate the attendant's mind. *I will stare at him with a merciful face; he will feel my mercy and offer me the same.* I tried to catch his gaze in the window, but he was looking off into space. Instead of using noise to grab his attention, I concentrated my immeasurably powerful mind on making him face me.

I finally caught his eye, but my attempts to manipulate his will were futile. He just shook his head back and forth as if to say *Man, you don't get it. You're going to be here all day.* My Zen gave way to panic again, and I began slamming my head against the walls. I wanted to scare him, to make him feel obligated to bring someone else in who could make a new evaluation. He wasn't impressed. I guess that's the point of the rubber in a rubber room. I took to the mat again and resumed crying until I had a banging headache and passed out.

The next morning I was back in my room when the Bird magically appeared. "Bird! When did you get here?"

"Just after midnight. I flew back from Chicago when Granny told me you were in the hospital."

I had so much to catch her up on. "Get me a pen and paper, now. I have to write some stuff down."

The Bird, never without a notebook and pen, handed them over.

"I need to make a list."

"Go ahead, honey."

I began scribbling furiously and produced the following list:

Things That Need to Happen

1. The Producer must masturbate
2. I have all the money in the world that I need
3. No crime is committed willfully
4. I'm a lawyer and a comedian
5. Some form of reparations / do something about gender inequality
6. Never do I get an STD
7. I want to write this list again tomorrow
8. Improve socioeconomic status of everyone

I handed my list over to the Bird and waited patiently while she looked it over. I thought that the key to my liberation lay in this list, and I was sure the Bird would concur.

"I'm not sure that all these make sense, Zack."

"Just because you don't understand them doesn't mean they don't make sense. I need to add one: 'No matter what, you can never let me shave my back hair.' Write that one down as number nine."

The Bird scribbled it down as if she'd just remembered she needed to pick up eggs from the grocery store.

"I have a…What do they call it when people get the wounds of Christ on their hands and feet? Or like when someone sees the Virgin Mary in a doughnut?"

"Stigmata."

"Right, stigmata. I have one of those in my back hair. The Virgin Mary is in my back hair. Therein lies my power."

"I'm not sure the Virgin Mary is in your back hair, son." Without arguing further, the Bird felt around for the outer edges of my crazy and tried to gently nudge me toward reality.

"It's there. You just can't see it. When did you first learn about Jesus?"

"You're feeling very spiritual today. I need you to do something for me, okay?"

"I will do my best." The tone of the dutiful son, treating his mother's words with biblical reverence.

"I need you to not run down the halls anymore. The staff told me that they had to put you in seclusion. I don't want you to be in seclusion."

"Well, I *look* out of control because I'm so fast—they're clearly not used to seeing a human with that sort of speed. I can run like an NFL cornerback."

"Please, just stop running. Think about your Granny. What would she say if she knew you were doing that?"

"*Zachariah!* Maybe pinch me."

"That's right. So think of your Granny."

"I will do my best. You know, I really don't want to die. I don't want to be in a box. But I accept that I am going to die in here. They're going to carry me out of here in a box." I wasn't Jesus per se, but with the Virgin Mary in my back hair and my new powers, I was definitely at least a prophet, and martyrdom seemed plausible.

"You aren't going to die, honey. You're going to get better."

Day 4 Good Shepherd (12/30/10)

Z crying for long spells / prays both Muslim and Christian. Toilet paper all over the floor of his room. Towels in the trash can. Looks worse than he did at Bellevue. "FALL RISK" yellow armband. He believes that the heater hisses when he says anything that hints at blasphemy. Nurse says, "He's asleep on his feet."

Day 6 Good Shepherd (1/1/11)

Z on fluid restrictions because he is drinking "pitchers" of water, according to the nurses — they think he is trying to flush out his medication. Taking shower after shower, often with his clothes on, bc he says that he's "done a lot of bad things and the showers cleanse me in more than just a physical way."

Day 7 Good Shepherd (1/2/11)

UNDER CONSTANT OBSERVATION. Jarhead orderly sits on folding chair outside of Z's room. Yesterday overheard him call Z "that asshole from NY." Told him not to talk about my son. "I don't know who your son is." / "He's the asshole from NY."

Day 9 Good Shepherd (1/4/11)

Turned the water in his room off. Flooded the bathroom. Nurses say it doesn't make sense that he's still psychotic. Gary is new caretaker — very patient and good with Zack. Z thinks he is God because his name starts with "G."

Day 10 Good Shepherd (1/5/11)

Random statements:
1. "I want to run like Forrest Gump."
2. "I'll make a Chewbacca noise." (and then does)

They escorted me out of building tonight because I refused to leave. "He's so much better when you're here," and then they kick me out. *My fears:* That he not snap out of it, that he be sent to a state hospital, that he not be able to be an attorney again.

To demonstrate the immense power of my mind, I'd started performing headstands in the sitting room. *This is what extreme concentration and meditation look like.* "Can you do this?" I would taunt my least favorite nurse, before wiping out.

"No, but I'm not a mental patient either," she would snap back.

"I can transcend you. None of you can control my mind. I am doing this through meditation alone. I don't even do yoga." My tumbling routines led to additional imposed seclusion: the rubber room became my pied-à-terre.

Of greater concern to the staff was my new party trick: wandering the halls completely naked. Even in front of my mother, I'd strip down completely naked and walk around my room.

"Zack! You have to keep your clothes on! They are going to send you to a state hospital!"

Around that time I also decided that it was time to go. Escape seemed easier here than at Bellevue, if for no other reason than we were on the first floor. At the end of the ward's main hall there was a nurses' station with a slick tile floor. If I could sprint through the station and make it out the other side, I could get within twenty feet of an unlocked door that led into the parking lot. Running through the nurses' station would be easy enough, but there was always a security guard standing at the hospital exit. The security guard was built like a pit bull. He had a military flattop: one guard on the sides, two guard on top. I got the impression that he'd welcome a confrontation. And yet, how much attention could he possibly be paying to an inactive exit?

Plenty of attention, as it turned out. I stood as close to the prohibitive yellow line as the rules allowed. This was probably my first mistake, as patients only approached the station when they wanted something—a snack, a Nicorette, missed medication. "What do you want?" the nurse on duty asked.

"Nothing, just looking."

"Why don't you go sit in the common area?"

"Yeah, I'm about to." *Fuck, did I blow my cover?* I decided they couldn't possibly suspect that I'd make a break for it after so obviously telegraphing my intentions. This was the stealing-beer-from-a-gas-station-by-slowly-walking-out-of-the-store technique: the clerk always pauses for a moment because he can't believe what he's seeing; the pause is enough to get out the doors, *then* you break into a sprint once you're in the parking lot.

I took a half step back from the line and looked away from the exit, hoping to throw them off the scent. *Okay, pussy, no more hesitation. One...two...three!* I got a good jump and, approaching my top speed, dropped to my knees in an attempt to get under the arms of the guard. I figured my unconventional approach might wrong-foot him. No such luck. The guard closed in on me fast, bent his knees and exploded into me, wrapping me up with such force that I thought I was being tased. "No! No! No!" he yelled. His form was perfect, his follow-through powerful and prolonged. He carried me all the way back across the prohibitive yellow line. "Get off of me! Get off me, you fuck! Fucking fascist!"

"I think we know where you're going!"

"You love that too, fake fucking pig!"

I squirmed out of his grasp and walked away, hoping not to give him a reason to manhandle me further. It didn't seem like he'd need much of a reason—*I was forced to engage and restrain the individual.* As for me, I did know where I was going: straight to isolation.

Day 12 Good Shepherd (1/7/11)

Wednesday at 5 p.m. Zack is placed in seclusion. 8 p.m. Zack is placed in restraints.

Day 13 Good Shepherd (1/8/11)

He thinks Sacha Baron Cohen is here.

Day 15 Good Shepherd (1/10/11)

Nurse says while Zack was in the gym playing catch with a security guard, he hit the guard in the face with a softball. Z says it was accidental.

After the softball incident, the staff started pushing harder to send me to Osawatomie State Hospital. "This is a short-term facility," they insisted. "He's not getting better. The drugs aren't working. He's been psychotic for more than two weeks." They told the Bird it was time to pursue "a more aggressive treatment route."

"I do not, under any circumstances, want him going to a state hospital." Her brother had spent the last fifteen years of his life in a state institution. She'd seen what those places looked like—dilapidated, underfunded, and understaffed; her brother in a straightjacket. "He is not going there."

They offered one final option: ECT, electroconvulsive therapy. Electric currents would be shot through my brain, intentionally triggering a brief seizure. Sometimes ECT can quickly reverse symptoms of certain mental illnesses. The hope was I'd just snap out of it. They showed her a video—it was a VHS from the 1980s.

"You will not be doing that to my son."

Once the Osawatomie talk resurfaced, she began bringing a photo of me to the hospital, like she'd done on her Bellevue visits. "That guy you are seeing is *not* my son. My son is sweet and empathetic. He's a feminist. He's not disrespectful to women. This isn't him," she said, clutching the picture. But they were done with me and she knew it. The nurses acknowledged that the guy in the picture looked much different from the strung-out lunatic who verbally abused them every day. They just couldn't reconcile that image with the man they were forced to care for. As far as they were concerned, the nice guy was *gone* and they wanted the crazy asshole who'd replaced him to be someone else's problem.

Day 17 Good Shepherd (1/12/11)

Judge court ordered Z to Osawatomie State Hospital. Left Good Shepherd at 11:30 a.m. Z out of nowhere tells me he wants to contact and make amends w/ father! Worthless sperm donor, doesn't even know his son is in a psych ward. Help me Jesus.

CHAPTER 17

I DIDN'T KNOW IT at the time, but it took a court order for the Bird to put us on a plane to California to visit our dad those summers. On the day of the custody and visitation hearing, Mack wore four shades of green to the Sedgwick County Courthouse: emerald-green suit jacket with mismatched forest-green slacks, a lime-green shirt, and a pine-green tie. And he slicked his hair back. He brought his mom with him to the proceedings. The Bird told the judge that, plain and simple, he didn't deserve to see his children. The judge agreed. "No, he doesn't. *But* they deserve to see him." So ordered. Summers in Cali.

No, he doesn't, but they do. Forget *seeing* him, I still wanted to *be* him at that point—I missed him tucking me in, Crown Royal on his breath or not. "Your whiskers tickle, Daddy." How could his face look so smooth and scratch so hard? And he played the drums. As far as musical instruments go, that's about as cool as it gets.

I felt like a man when he let me hang out with him. Before he left, the proudest day of my life had been when we'd demolished the concrete steps on the side of our house on Laura Street with sledgehammers. The sledgehammer I used weighed half as much as me, and it brought me tumbling backward the first time I swung it over my head. But I didn't want to choke up on the handle; I wanted to chop down on it, like Paul Bunyan splitting logs. Like my dad was doing.

It was hot, and as workingmen do, we took our shirts off. My mom brought us hot dogs and purple Kool-Aid, and we ate and drank outside. That part felt manly too: the womenfolk bringing out provisions. The only thing that could have made it better was if we'd worn hard hats like real construction workers. He smoked pot and drank Crown and Cokes throughout the workday. I didn't know it was pot then, but once I was old enough to have friends who smoked, I recognized the smell immediately: childhood. It smelled like his friend Billy's velour couch; it smelled like when he was in a good mood; it smelled like those demolished steps.

Before our first summer visit to see Mack, California was only a concept to me—like the rain forest or Antarctica. I was aware of its existence but only as an amalgamation of clichés ripped from TV and magazine covers. L.A. meant surfer dudes, Disneyland, the Hollywood Walk of Fame, blondes, and the Lakers. And the beach—I didn't associate with anyone who'd ever seen the Pacific Ocean, except maybe Pa during his military service. Cool-guy ambitions of all sorts revealed themselves as possibilities. Would I learn to surf? I started weaving "I'm going to L.A. to see my dad this summer" into conversations in the Kellogg Elementary School cafeteria.

It being 1990, and me being seven, Mom and Granny accompanied us to the gate. While I watched the planes take off, Granny gripped my hand with misbehaving-in-church-level pressure. Giant sharks with wings, longer than a soccer field and taller than my house. I knew they weren't fighter jets, but I imagined where the guns would be positioned. (They'd blast out of the turbines.) Every pilot strolling through the terminal was Goose; no Mavericks, sadly. But 300 miles per hour! We were about to blast through the sky at 300 miles per hour! I expected it to feel something like a space shuttle launch. I couldn't wait to watch *Top Gun* with my dad again. It seemed like he watched it every night when he lived with us—I'd pretend I couldn't sleep so that he'd let me lie on the couch next to him.

The Bird tried to wear a brave face, but she couldn't hold it in any longer when the gate attendant called for all unaccompanied minors to board. Alexa cried too, which made me cry; Adam was too young to join in. He just clutched his stuffed Littlefoot doll—he'd watched *The Land Before Time* so many times that he broke the VHS tape. My sister's tears sprang from understanding where we were headed; mine were solely on account of leaving my mom and Granny. I'd never spent twenty-four hours away from the Bird, and now we'd be gone for the summer. We'd be taller the next time she saw us. "Take care of your brothers," the Bird said, holding Alexa tight.

Mack drove like a goddamn maniac. Left lane, right lane, left lane, back to the right, yelling "Get your head out of your ass!"—or some variation thereof—the entire time. It was hilarious to me, and for some reason not at all terrifying. "Get your head out of your ass!" What a phenomenal turn of phrase. Every driver on the 405 was "This idiot." Alexa gripped the dashboard and sighed audibly as Mack darted in and out of the idiots. "Can we get something to eat, Dad?"

"Yeah, honey. But first, welcome to Hollywood!" He said it like he owned the place.

He took us to Red Robin. It was as nice as any restaurant I'd ever set foot inside. *Excuse me, am I reading this menu correctly? Does that say* unlimited *french fries? Keep 'em coming then, miss.*

"If I was homeless, I'd come here every day in the morning and stay all day and eat french fries."

"Just eat your food."

My mom would have been impressed with such a cunning plan.

After Red Robin, Mack went out of his way to drive us by the Hollywood sign. "It used to say 'Hollywoodland'!" That sounded dumb to me. "Hollywood" was so much punchier—maybe that's why they'd changed it. And maybe the reason he was taking us on such a jaunt—wining and dining and french-frying us, showing off the iconic Hollywood landscape—was that our destination was not truly Hollywood, or even L.A. at large; it was Cerritos, a suburb in Los Angeles County. There were Targets and liquor stores and Chinese massage parlors next to insurance offices in strip malls. Where was the ocean? The surfers? Where was Tom Cruise?

California quickly revealed itself to be a series of semi-adventures we couldn't afford. Alexa, ten, was the first to point this out. We ate out almost every night for dinner—at Sizzler or Souplantation! or Red Robin. (Occasionally at Cracker Barrel; never at the Medieval Times across the street from Cracker Barrel, although promises were made.) An average bill would run about $50, and most dinners were paid for by Maggie—Mack's new girlfriend—who had a job at Sony. Mack very occasionally pulled editing work at a local news station during that first summer we visited, but his jobs were few and far between. I knew he didn't have any money because Alexa knew he didn't have any money. She'd beg Mack, "Can't we just eat peanut butter and jelly sandwiches tonight? I'll make them."

"My dinner doesn't come on two pieces of bread," Mack told her.

The restaurant experiences were mortifying. He always flirted with the waitresses, even in front of Maggie, who would later become his second wife. Usually, we ate at name-tag places, so he could just look at the server's chest to get her name. He'd then address her for the rest of dinner like they were old pals from college, either by first name or "hun," which he most often slipped in at least once.

The overt flirtation was only the second most embarrassing thing about going out to eat with him. Motivated by both gluttony and poverty, he'd always ask the waitress, "Can we get a few more of these rolls, boxed up to go?" He carried himself as if he were some sort of bread connoisseur. "They're just so good. I'd love to take a few of those rolls home. Can't beat those rolls." Maybe it was because I knew we actually needed to take the bread home (he wasn't above eating his *lunch* on two pieces of bread), but his affected nonchalance made it seem obvious that he was hiding a certain shame in his request. He'd even continue the front with us after our waitress left the table: "This really is good bread. Isn't this good bread?" Yes, they are rolls. Rolls with butter are good.

Restaurants weren't our only luxury. We saw pretty much every movie that came out. Once we worked through the first-run titles, we hit the dollar theaters. There was less tension in the air at the buck flicks. No Alexa saying, "Three kids is fifteen dollars, two adults is sixteen dollars, that's thirty-one. Plus, you always get popcorn and two big Cokes, so that's another seventeen dollars, which makes the total forty-eight."

"You can't go to a movie without popcorn," Mack would scold. Mack liked his popcorn prepared a very specific way. When the concessions employee would ask him "Butter?" he'd always answer with "Butter layered throughout." No matter how many times he had to explain it, he refused to acknowledge that his request was unorthodox. He couldn't wait for them to ask so that he could offer his explanation: "You pour some popcorn in the bucket, then a layer of butter. Then layer of popcorn…layer of butter. One more popcorn scoop. Then, you guessed it, layer of butter. Repeat until full." He thought it was funny; a second grader could tell it was condescending. Mack would then turn to us, shake his head, and roll his eyes, as if to say *Can you believe these idiots? Never heard of butter throughout.* Alexa and I learned to silently apologize to all manner of service industry workers, with shoulder shrugs, pursed smiles, and eyebrow pops. *It's not you, it's him.* The popcorn was so goddamn oily with that fake butter-flavored canola oil that it became an amorphous solid and never failed to give me a stomachache. I couldn't stop eating it, though.

After the movie, Mack always stayed until the last credit rolled.

"Huh, Greg Calvin worked on this," he'd mutter to himself and all of us. "Anne Schneider." Maggie pretended to believe that he knew some of these people.

If asked what he did for a living, Mack answered, "I'm a producer, director, and editor." Sometimes, casually, "I work in television" or "I'm in show business." In reality, Dad was a man who needed to get his head out of his ass. In his more grounded moods he'd say as much, and he would plan to do so. That's how he started most phone conversations: "I'm about to get my head out of my ass." Soon, tomorrow, next week, he would. You got the sense that, to this man, pulling one's head out of one's ass was an exquisitely complicated procedure.

To his children, the solution seemed simpler. Every summer we begged him to get a job — anywhere. When we'd go to Red Robin in the Cerritos Mall, Alexa would slyly read the NOW HIRING sign aloud. Eventually, we just started begging him outright:

"Why don't you get a job at Red Robin?"

"I don't wait tables."

"Why don't you get a job at Best Buy?"

"They don't make any money."

"They make more than zero money."

"I work in Hollywood."

"Home Depot?"

"I don't work for minimum wage. My work is in Hollywood."

In 2007, the summer before my final year of law school, I visited my dad in California for the last time. It had been ten years since I'd last been out there, and I'd probably seen him in person five times since. Nothing had changed.

After working on his cars and smoking pot at his shop all day, we retreated to his apartment. Sure as the ground beneath our feet, his wife teetered over, blackout drunk, slurring and pretending she wasn't. My brother, sister, and I learned of Maggie's alcoholism live and in color one summer afternoon twelve years prior while we were watching Maury Povich — our third consecutive hour of daytime talk shows — waiting for Mack to take us to McDonald's. From upstairs, we heard Mack yell, "If you love it so much, why don't you wear it!?" Followed by the unmistakable gasp of someone who'd had vodka thrown on their person. Then one of them threw something that hit the wall. We muted *Maury;* this was better. "CAPTAIN FUCKING SNEAK-A-DRINK!" Mack yelled.

"You fucking threw my drink on me!" Maggie confirmed what we already knew. "Fucking, fuck. Bastard!"

A couple of minutes later, Mack sauntered downstairs, easy as Sunday morning, and casually asked us, "You guys want to go see a movie?" We did.

Maggie didn't.

Later that night, Mack ignored Captain Sneak-a-Drink and started picking my brain about my upcoming legal career possibilities.

"Will you be my lawyer?"

"What do you mean?"

"Would you represent me?"

Of course I knew literally what "Will you be my lawyer?" meant, but it didn't seem my unemployed father was presently in need of representation. And I was a second-year law student, specializing in criminal law. "Why?" I asked. "Are you thinking about committing a crime?" Best-case scenario, he meant parking tickets.

He pointed to the TV. We were watching *Ocean's Twelve.* "No, I mean, like, if I produced *Ocean's Thirteen,* would you represent me?"

Fuck. I felt the heat rising from my collarbone and into my skull. I tried not to answer too quickly, but I didn't want to pause too long either. Don't say it. Don't say it. Don't say: *What, are you just going to* call George and say "Let's call Brad, get the gang back together—do it with me. Fuck Steven Soderbergh. I'll shoot it in my garage." I didn't say it, but I couldn't just leave it either.

"Do you really think you could produce *Ocean's Thirteen*?" I asked.

"Why not?" Silence.

You know why not, motherfucker. You didn't do Ocean's Twelve, *or* Eleven. *Your alcoholic wife is standing in the kitchen, too drunk to make couscous. You are drinking MGD. Your only computer weighs thirty-five pounds and you don't have the internet. Your last "project" was a "commercial" for toner cartridge refills, and they didn't turn out to be the wave of the future you were predicting. You don't have health insurance. You don't own a cell phone. You just smoked your seventh Marlboro Ultra Light in forty-five minutes. The baseball-pitching machine you bought me when I was twelve is still in its box in your garage. You have three cars on cinder blocks, no checking account, and you bum weed from your next-door neighbor. You are not producing* Ocean's Thirteen, Fourteen, *or* Fifty-seven.

"Like, if I get my head out of my ass and produce *Ocean's Thirteen*, would you represent me?" He wasn't at all kidding.

Goddammit…

"Sure, I'll represent you. That'd be a nice commission. I wouldn't know how to do it, but I'd figure it out."

"You'd figure it out!"

I accidentally broke my first Mack rule: quit trying to impress your father.

After I agreed to be his lawyer, Mack had one more favor to ask: "You have to tell me the secret after they swear you in."

"The what?"

"The secret. When they swear you into the bar, there's a secret they tell all lawyers."

"Is that right?" Shooting down conspiracy theories without coming across as condescending is difficult. Also, with Mack, entertaining his fixations can become a "choose your own adventure." Challenge the lawyer theory and he'd just move on to the next one, about health care or rigged elections or sex offenders or the politics of Hollywood or Jesus or the Bible or... take your pick.

"Sure, I'll tell you." We clinked our MGD cans on it.

CHAPTER 18

SACHA BARON COHEN WAS being transferred from Good Shepherd along with me in the van. Our destination was B2 — the violent and sexual offenders ward at Osawatomie State Hospital. Good Shepherd reported that I met *both* criteria: violent from the softball incident, sexual from my nudist walks.

Even filtered through the gloomy gray glaze of winter, the farms and fence posts dotting the Kansas plains looked idyllic. The landscape seemed so slow — the polar opposite of my brain. If I could just get out of the van, I could run through those fields to the end of the earth, no locked doors between us. Had I known what hell awaited me, I would have tried harder.

Osawatomie State Hospital is two hours and several decades away from Wichita. Set in the middle of the flat Kansas prairie, it was originally built in 1855 and known then as the Kansas Insane Asylum — folks preferred plain-speak back in those days, before we started pretending loony bins were hospitals. Owing to a ghost infestation, the original structure had to be destroyed long ago, but if the original had been knocked down on account of a few poltergeists, it's hard to say why the 1970s replacement has thus far been spared the wrecking ball. When I walked in, the original linoleum was peeling and stained, the drinking fountain appeared to be duct-taped to the wall, and the fluorescent lights, those that worked, cast a stale glow over the place.

By the time I got to Osawatomie, I was still having starbursts of psychosis, but lucidity was slowly returning in patches. That said, I didn't give my state of affairs much thought: I was so heavily medicated that it didn't occur to me to think about where I'd been for the past couple of weeks.

An old man walked around the common area with his pants dropped well below his bare ass. He was stroking his cock but no one really seemed to mind. He looked like he'd been living in a shack in the woods plotting against the government for several years: coarse, scraggly gray hair, beard to match, decaying brown and yellow teeth. Finally an orderly told him to put it away. He mumbled something guttural, sounding incapable of regular speech.

"Monk Monk! Monk Monk! Monk Monk!" A chiseled beast of a man—six foot five, 240 pounds at least—was roaming the halls and yelling "Monk Monk! Have you met Monk Monk?" over and over again. He got in the faces of fellow patients who were either indifferent or too terrified to tell him to fuck off. That he was speaking in a six-year-old's voice made him even *more* terrifying—a six-year-old with a silverback's size and strength.

As soon as he noticed me, he sped over and started in with the Monk Monk routine. "Monk Monk. This is Monk Monk. I'm Gregory and this is Monk Monk. Say hi to Monk Monk." His pupils were dilated and pinballing back and forth inside his eye sockets. Even a crazy could tell he was fucking crazy. I figured I'd better say hi to Monk Monk.

In a high-pitched voice, the stuffed monkey perched on his shoulder said hi back. "Give Monk Monk a kiss," commanded Gregory, utterly childlike in his glee.

I kissed Monk Monk.

"You're gorgeous, you know that?"

"Thanks," I muttered.

"I could have a lot of fun with you."

"I think we'll be keeping it platonic, if it's all the same."

Gregory laughed hard and continued to Monk Monk around the room.

I noticed on my first trip to the bathroom that there were unattended group showers here. Not to mention we were on the ward for *violent and sexual offenders*. Which was Gregory? Which would I even prefer him to be? Or was he both? I looked up and saw the second masturbator of the day. This one was sweating heavily and quietly groaning with pleasure.

The Bird drove to Osawatomie the next morning and checked into a motel that shared a parking lot with a Pizza Hut and a liquor store. The carpeting crackled and was sticky if she stepped on it barefoot. There was a wobbly table with a mini fridge, which she moved onto the floor so she could use her laptop there. The water in the toilet rose nearly all the way to the lid when flushed, and the DO NOT DISTURB sign had a Band-Aid stuck to it. But the motel was one exit from the hospital—that's all that really mattered.

The Bird told the owner, a middle-aged man from India, that her son was sick and in the hospital, and that she couldn't afford to pay $45 per night. She told him $40 was the most she could pay, and he told her no way. "I'll just have to leave tomorrow, then," she said. When she got to the room, he called and said that $40 would be okay. He would lose money, but he would do it for her. He told her that his wife "stay in India," and he was a teacher and had a son who was a doctor. She told him that she was a teacher too and that her son was a lawyer.

On the drive to the hospital, she spoke with Dr. Singh. After my sixteen days of psychosis, he was coming around to the view that a more aggressive approach might be warranted. She made it just in time to line up early for visiting hours.

An African American orderly with a thick Kansas twang walked me down the corridor and led me to the visiting room. I was the only patient with a visitor. She followed me into the room and sat on a metal folding chair in the corner. No unsupervised visits.

I could barely lift my head, but I knew I was in the violent and sexual offenders ward. The screams rattling off the walls of the ward were constant and horrifying. Their distance made them more unsettling — without a visual, the imagination was free to suspect the worst. And like a pack of coyotes, the howls of one would ignite a chain reaction, the pack instinctually set off by its own energy. Terror, on a fucking loop. Psychosis doesn't shield you from fear. "You gotta get me out of here," I kept telling her. "You gotta get me outta here."

In between visits, she was either power walking (when there wasn't a blizzard), working at the makeshift desk in her motel room, or going to Walmart. Unlike at Bellevue, we were permitted a few of life's creature comforts at Osawatomie, but they had to be shipped. So the Bird would go to Walmart and buy beef jerky, Doritos, Snickers, candy, and juice, then mail them to me. The provisions were crucial, as the food was awful at OSH — even worse than at Bellevue. Since no one else got care packages, I shared my spoils with the other charges of the state. A "first to ask, first served" policy seemed fairest. The inmates devoured everything, especially the candy. Altruism aside, my generosity served me well. I was like a mob boss in prison. You want the Snickers, you don't fuck with me. You try to fuck with me, I got plenty of folks on my Snickers payroll.

The Bird sometimes shopped for herself as well. At the Dollar General, townies would stare her down for wearing slimmish jeans, even though they were from Walmart. In her motel room she read journal articles about black males in alternative education programs. Between my two hospitalizations and the death of her fake husband, she'd fallen well behind on her PhD research. Graduation would have to wait another year.

During the Bird's second visit, an orderly told her, "No one ever leaves this unit." The Bird was again the only visitor. That's the other thing: "No one gets visitors here. Sometimes we go months without seeing anyone. No one cares. They don't have anyone. Some of these people have been here for years and never had a visitor."

I may have been the Gorilla, but Gregory was King Kong of that motherfucker. Anyone else could have walked around with a spiked club in hand and you'd prefer it to Gregory wandering the halls shirtless with his stuffed monkey resting atop his shoulder. Fights were common on the ward, but no one stepped to Gregory. The staff kept their distance as well, and he was eager to tell me why.

"I was a Navy SEAL. And I'm a black belt. Nobody can restrain me here. When they try, they have big problems."

Normally, an infantilized giant living in a psych ward with a stuffed monkey best friend would be at the top of my probably-not-a-Navy-SEAL list. But Gregory reminded me of my high school friend Lance—a Green Beret, aikido and knives expert, top of his class in physical conditioning at West Point—only bigger. I believed him.

"Can you show me some moves? Like, don't hurt me, but show me how to fend off an attack?"

"Oh yeah." If a laugh can be calmly maniacal, that's the sound he made.

"But don't hurt me, okay? Nice and slow."

"Won't hurt you. Too pretty."

"Okay, so I throw a punch." I slowly directed my fist toward his face. "And you…"

"Grab wrist." He did. "Rotate counterclockwise." He did. "Shatter nose with left hand." He didn't.

Even in slow motion, his fluidity and power revealed how effortlessly this man could break me. I was sure he wouldn't even need his hands — he could roundhouse kick my face off. But, also like Lance, he was gentle; he stopped when I said "Stop." If he understood nothing else, he seemed to understand his own strength.

He clearly enjoyed demonstrating his talents, but he'd also confirmed he was a trained killing machine. Sure, he liked me now, but what if that switch flipped? What if the thing that had landed him in here was a propensity to attack people he's close to? Like a kid getting riled up before bedtime, he wasn't entirely in possession of his impulses. The maniacally calm smile never exploded into full-on hysterics, but it simmered, slow and steady.

Osawatomie was not only a state hospital, but it also housed criminal defendants who'd been found not guilty by reason of insanity. I discovered this when I asked a young Hispanic patient what he was in for.

"Murder," he said. I waited for a laugh or some indication that it was just the crazy talking. "Double murder."

"You're fucking serious? Wow."

"It's fucked-up. Yeah. I killed two people. I was young. I had a drug problem."

"So you have to stay here forever? Or they can only hold you until you're no longer a danger to yourself or others?"

"That's right. It will probably be a couple of years."

He was short and baby faced. It was impossible to imagine him killing one person, let alone two. Did he shoot them? Hammer? Stab? Choke? Stabbed seemed most likely — it just lined up with the psych ward element. Shooting requires a certain coordination and skill, no one carries a hammer with them, and it would be hard to strangle two people at once. Stabbed. Had to be stabbed. I told him I didn't judge him. There was nothing wrong with staying on the murderer's good side. But I meant it too. People always ask public defenders how we can defend people we know are guilty. One of many reasons for me is that I don't believe too strongly in the existence of choice. Nobody wants to be fucked-up.

* * *

Although there was no shortage of screamers or fighters, many of the patients at Osawatomie bordered on comatose. The two masturbators lacked vigor; sometimes it seemed they weren't even conscious of the fact they were jerking off in a crowded, semipublic space. It was hard to determine how our dosages were calculated. Was the staff actually *aiming* for comatose? The default was clearly to err on the side of *over*medicating. From a liability standpoint, it made sense: should a patient (say, Gregory) lose control and become violent, the hospital would be open to lawsuits. But what are the damages if a patient is overmedicated? The cost of a load of laundry to clean up the drool on his shirt?

My overmedication had messier consequences. Going back on Depakote introduced a level of constipation I'd never known existed. After three days without being able to shit, I could barely walk. My abdomen felt like it was full of concrete. We had to go to the nurses' station for any medical needs, minor or otherwise. Headache? Need permission to take a Tylenol. And so I had to explain to the attendant what I was going through.

"I need something," I pleaded, holding my stomach.

"What you need, man?"

"I can't shit. Haven't shit for days. I can barely move."

"I can give you some Milk of Magnesia."

Milk of Magnesia sounded like something you'd purchase from an apothecary.

"This is gonna work?" I asked him.

"It should. If it don't, come back, man."

"I need this to work. I am suffering. Really."

He handed me a plastic shot glass and I threw back the sweet, chalky substance.

"Now what?"

"Wait twenty or thirty."

"You serious? You don't have something that works quicker? This is an issue here."

"You gotta try this first."

I waited the twenty. Nothing. I tried to quit thinking about it, but the discomfort was rapidly increasing. I asked for something else. He poured me another shot of Milk of Magnesia.

"You sure I can't just chug that whole thing?"

"I know you in pain, man. Just wait a little bit."

Ten more minutes and I was back at the medication desk. This time I just shook my head.

He opened a different drawer and pulled out a plastic bullet that looked like half a glue stick for a glue gun. "You put this in your rectum. It should work." I waddled down the hall, wondering why we hadn't pursued the "should work" option first.

In the bathroom, I sat in the community stall and pushed the glycerin bullet up my butt. It hurt a little. Hoping to take my mind off my excruciating discomfort, I decided to take a shower while the bullet worked its magic.

You'd think it would be impossible to shit yourself while standing eight feet away from a toilet, especially when you're already completely naked. You'd be wrong. In my defense, I was not given sufficient warning regarding this product's efficacy. My body skipped entirely the moment of *Go, now. Drop everything you are doing and run or walk, whichever gives you the best chance, to the nearest bathroom or open field.* Skipped right over it. I exploded. Like a fire hydrant. All over the shower floor. It was one of the most embarrassing and relieving moments of my life. Luckily, even if I had been caught in the act, I'd never been around a peer group I cared less about impressing. Who was going to judge me, the hallway masturbators?

Still, I am a human and my primordial instincts kicked in to tell me, *Clean this up and get the fuck out of here.* Even a dog kicks some dirt behind him after he does his business. I was ill-equipped to erase the entire crime scene, so I just tried to get myself clean and dressed in under sixty seconds, all the while praying no one would come in. Miraculously, I got away with it.

Or so I thought. Upon exiting the bathroom, the obvious move was to walk to the complete opposite end of the ward. Then I'd casually mill about, at a safe distance, of course, but close enough to hear any shrieks of discovery. Minutes later, what I saw instead was a janitor walking down the hall with the official industrial yellow mop bucket. "Feeling better?" he asked as we passed each other in the hall. I looked at the ground and mumbled "Yeah" in a tone that I hoped conveyed *I can neither confirm nor deny.*

For some of us, B2 was a prison; for others, it was home. One evening, after the customary "Monk Monk!" salutation, Gregory invited me back to his room. "I have some stuff I need to show you," he said, as he fished a shoebox full of mementos out of his dresser. "You see that, it says 'Langley.'" He displayed what looked to be a legit photo ID. "I'm ex-CIA," he said. "Well, actually," he corrected himself, "I *am* CIA. Once in, never out. I'm an expert in hand-to-hand combat, scuba missions, explosives, and covert ops. I'm Rambo," he told me. "Feel my head—right there…" He grabbed my hand and placed it on top of his skull. "Right there. You feel that? Knock on it." I gently tapped it. "No, go ahead, really knock on it." I gave it a knock. "I have a metal plate in my head." It felt hard enough to be plausible. Then he showed me scars on his torso where he'd been stabbed, and discussed his high body count and the methods he'd used to achieve it—sniper rifle, knife, helicopter gunner. "Oh, and I'm an eighth-degree black belt."

Then he grabbed my belly, shook it like he was playing with a baby, and roared like a lion. "RAAARRRRR!" That crazy-ass laugh started bubbling to the surface again. His kettle seemed to always run just a little below boiling. "Monk Monk! Monk Monk! Monk Monk misses you!"

"I'm right here, Monk Monk. Chill."

Then he was right back to telling stories about killing jihadists in various Middle Eastern countries. "Oh, and *this* box—this is what I need to show you. You live in New York, right? You recognize that?"

"No." It was a photograph of a giant mansion.

"That's Connecticut."

"Okay."

"That's my family's house. I am super, super, super fucking rich."

"Why do you live here?"

"Have you heard of Random House?"

"Yeah."

"My family *owns* it. We are billionaires."

"Random House makes you a billionaire?"

"Look at that house!"

"It's nice."

"Do you know how much I could pay you for a blowjob?" he asked, with a hint of maniacal laughter.

"Well, a lot, I guess."

"You're smart."

"Let me ask you a question." I figured now was as good a time as any to switch gears. "Have they ever had to take you down in here—shoot you full of tranq darts?"

"Ohhhh yeah! Oh yeah!" His face lit up. "First they sent three security guards. I took all of them out. Then they called the police and they tried to storm in. I took all six of them out. Then they brought in the sheriffs with rubber bullets and shot me up. It took several rounds to get me to the ground. Then I grabbed on to the drinking fountain. I ripped it off the wall! They finally got on top of me and hog-tied my ankles to my wrists." He gestured toward the water fountain outside his room. It looked sturdier than when I'd first regarded it. Of course I'd yet to consider what it might take to rip a water fountain out of the goddamn wall.

"I told you—I'm Rambo."

"I believe you."

Gregory and I sat together at most of our meals. Breakfast was served at 7:30 a.m. and it truly was the most important meal of the day—you can't fuck up cereal. In the evenings, Gregory wouldn't go to dinner without his expensive-looking, but old and shabby, houndstooth blazer. Occasionally I couldn't take his "Monk Monk!" and I sat by myself. But you're never truly alone in these places—personal space is a foreign concept to most, and certainly there is no expectation of privacy or peace and quiet. Screaming never becomes ambient; it's always screaming. We are biologically designed to be made uncomfortable by it—to be incapable of tolerating it, really. Our irritation is the only reason babies survive infancy.

After twenty-six days in the hospital, my sanity finally started to crystallize. It felt more like a fog lifting than a light switch flipping on. It was a double-edged sword. I began to see the ward for what it was—a dangerous place full of volatile patients sensitive to provocation. I started to spend nearly all my time in my room doing push-ups by the hundreds to calm myself.

The nurses at B2 continued telling the Bird that I didn't belong there. But she couldn't lobby for my release until I'd regained lucidity. As soon as she detected Zack returning in my eyes, she reminded me of what I needed to do: I wrote out a request to be discharged, affirming that I was not a danger to myself or others.

I got an exit interview with the head psychiatrist the next morning. Trying to establish early and unequivocally that I was of sound mind, I told him I was aware that I'd been in the throes of a psychotic break for twenty-six days now, and that I wasn't any longer. And then I asked him, "My mom says I might be borderline schiz. What does that mean?"

"That means each one of these episodes puts you at greater risk of having another. And the line between bipolar one and schizophrenia can be blurry. This episode lasted much longer than your previous. Each one blurs the line a little bit more. Marijuana…"

"No marijuana. I know."

"No marijuana. Ever. You don't react normally to it. It can trigger the psychosis."

He said he was keeping me on the Depakote for now, that I could talk to Dr. Singh about transitioning back to Lamictal when he thought it was safe. Until then, I had to stay on the Depakote. "You are vulnerable right now."

"I understand."

He set a discharge date for two days later and told me I had a wonderful mother.

CHAPTER 19

THE BIRD AND I gunned it out of town. I was glad to see Osawatomie recede in the rearview mirror, but I was terrified we'd one day be making this drive again. Or, worse, what if I only made a one-way trip—the drive there but never the drive back. After all, no one but me left while I was there.

"Hey," I told the Bird. "Would you ever let me live like Uncle Eddie?"

"No."

"Do you think Granny and Pa thought they'd let Uncle Eddie live like Uncle Eddie?"

"No."

"So do you think they had a choice?"

"No."

"So how can you know?... Don't ever fucking let me live like Uncle Eddie, okay? Don't ever let me be one of those people who never leaves. You promise me that?"

"Yes."

"Chain me to the fucking wall if you need to, but let me live in the basement."

Just because I understand the legal issues of a guardianship proceeding didn't mean I wouldn't one day be the subject of one. How many times could I wiggle out of this straightjacket before I drowned?

We stopped at a gas station fifty miles down the highway from Osawatomie. I shuffled in like an old man at a nursing home but came to life when I saw the hot dogs on the roaster—plump dogs, sweating and spinning hypnotically. They'd probably been there for hours, but they looked *so* delicious. I finished two and was working on a third before my mom even pumped the gas. When she came inside to pay, my fingers and beard were coated in ketchup. "No money," I tried to say, but my mouth was so full I was nearly choking. I pointed to the hot dog roller, held up three fingers, and pointed to the cash register. "No money. Pay him. I had three."

"I think that clerk thought you were extorting me," the Bird said when we were back on the highway.

Riding in the car while my mom drove felt like a relic of a bygone era. Were we going to soccer practice? To school? To the movies for a middle school date? I used to love having her all to myself in the car, and I had that same feeling now, like the car was our oasis. I felt safe. Our nightmare was over.

Speaking of nightmares, Mack McD was in the 'Ta when I got back. Other than the first couple of Christmases after he moved to California, Mack didn't visit Wichita much. He came after I was expelled in sixth grade and smacked me in the face after I said something smartass to him—something in the vein of "You want to come in here and act like a parent now? You're gonna set me straight?" The Bird told him she needed to speak with him in the basement and grabbed him by the collar. "You have no right!" she told him. "You have no idea what goes on here." He told her, "You're real tough, Cindy. I'll leave. I know I'm not welcome here."

Mack otherwise only came to town when he felt like he was obligated. Such obligations usually marked the end of an era of some sort—Alexa's senior violin recital, for example, or my senior soccer season. With these visits, there was usually accompanying praise to be accepted about what fine children he'd raised and how he must be so proud. "I am," he would say, or sometimes, "We are," like it was a team effort.

As far as high school soccer players go in Wichita, Kansas, I was pretty good—started varsity all four years, sat on the bench for one year at a Division I school. Which is all only to say that soccer was the most important thing in my life from ages six to nineteen. Mack always said he intended to come see a game or two, but freshman year turned into senior year quicker than he'd anticipated. In the fall of 2000, he realized it was now or never.

He flew to Wichita and immediately made his presence felt, overwhelmingly so. He started attending practices, made every game, and went to the social get-togethers the soccer moms organized. After games, he'd buy us beer and drink and smoke his ass off with us. Before long, he was a valued member of the Northwest Grizzlies soccer community. His gift to the team was to be a highlight reel that he'd shoot and edit himself. After all, he was a "producer, director, and editor" in Hollywood.

Mack scored the opening sequence of the highlight film to Kenny Loggins's "Highway to the Danger Zone" before transitioning to Stevie Ray Vaughan's rendition of "Voodoo Child." The choice of the latter track was in no way influenced by any consideration of the musical taste of the players on the team—Eminem and Linkin Park would otherwise have been best. Mack's song selection was instead all but an out-and-out declaration that he'd been through a pretty heavy cocaine period.

Despite having never purchased a pair of shin guards, Mack was recognized for his contribution at the end-of-season banquet. In fairness, he did put his best effort into the production. At the City League finals, he lay on his belly in the grass after persuading the three team captains to run out of the equipment shed before roster introductions so he could shoot their "playoff shoes" from the ground. As they burst through the barn door, he popped up off his belly and jogged with them to midfield, holding the camera at knee height all the way to the center circle.

The film was well received, but he still left the awards ceremony with a bad taste in his mouth. His intention, as it turns out, wasn't simply to create a highlight reel to give to the players and parents purely out of goodwill; he also aimed to turn a modest profit in the process. The DVDs were set up at the cafeteria's exit, with a box for cash next to the stack of discs. But the parents missed the cashbox and simply helped themselves to the DVDs, gratis. On the way to the party that followed the ceremony, he stated numerous times that he didn't really care, how that wasn't really the point anyway, and it wasn't about the money. But he continued to grumble under his breath, "They can have the fucking things. It's nice to get compensated for your time, but they can have the fucking things." Twenty minutes later, he was in Mrs. Searfoorce's basement, holding up her son by the legs while he set the evening's keg stand record.

I had no idea Mack was in Wichita when I left Osawatomie. Neither did the Bird. The bigger shock was that I'd apparently invited him. Lost to the hazy fog of lifting psychosis was the call I'd made from the pay phone at Osawatomie, asking him to come visit. My brother broke the news to me when the Bird and I got home. We hugged each other first. Then we cried.

"Are you okay, BB?"

"I'm okay, LB. Dark side of the moon. But I've been there before."

My brother told me that Mack had shown up the night before, stoned out of his mind. "He wants you to call him."

I did call him. I figured I was obliged to if I was indeed the only reason he'd flown into town. We made a lunch date for the next day. I wasn't 100 percent sure he'd make it.

My dad picked me up in his friend Drake's sun-bleached, primer-red '88 Pontiac Grand Am. It smelled like an ashtray—Drake owns a decent portion of the merchandise offered in the Marlboro Miles loyalty catalog. Mack was also blowing Marlboro Ultra Lights all the way to the restaurant. I told him to give me one and he handed me a cig, though he'd yet to say anything to me beyond "Hey" and "Where do you want to eat?"

We went through the Jason's Deli line in silence. Neither of us considered the salad bar. I took my usual: turkey wrap with avocado and baked Lay's. Mack ordered an open-face Reuben with regular chips and a Coke. *You are a fucking open-face Reuben,* I thought.

Once we sat down, I couldn't meet his eyes, but I could feel that he was staring straight at my forehead, ready to catch mine the second I looked up. When I finally did, his expression was exactly as I thought it would be: mouth agape with his big bottom lip protruding. The mouth breathing and the plump lips, combined with his wide-set eyes, made him look like a freshly caught sea bass. His eyebrows were raised, accentuating that big forehead of his; it's always a little bigger and a little more wrinkled every time I see him. I recognized the two middle wrinkles as recent additions to my own forehead. I closed my own big gaping lips and made a note to be more vigilant about mouth breathing. He looked pained as he tried to decide whether he was supposed to be here for support or discipline.

If he was waiting on me to break the silence, it was going to be a quiet Reuben. I wasn't giving him the cold shoulder for cold shoulder's sake, but I'd only seen him three times in the past four years: once at his mom's funeral, once at my sister's veterinary school graduation, and most recently at our *Ocean's Thirteen* "production meeting," after which he screamed at me for setting a pot of hot water on his countertop. "Don't put that there! There's no finish on the wood!" He'd been planning on finishing them for seventeen years. I walked away, he followed me, things escalated, and I ended up putting my fist through a wall. He grabbed me by the neck, cocked his fist in front of my face, and said, "I should knock you the fuck out!" Then he told me that "the little lion always wants to take down Mufasa." I laughed in his face, thinking (a) *This forty-seven-year-old man's worldview relies entirely too much on* The Lion King; *and* (b) *That's not even how the movie goes—Simba was destroyed by his father's death; it was Mufasa's brother, Scar, who orchestrated the hit.*

I told him the most painful thing I could think of: "You know what? You're right. Your kids do think you're a goddamn joke and we've thought you were a goddamn joke for a long time now." I felt stupid about that sooner than I expected since the next day I had to rely on him for a ride to the airport. We drove to LAX together in silence.

So there was catching up to do—more ground than we could cover over a fast-casual dining experience. And I didn't expect we'd ever discuss the psych ward or my mental health problems. I didn't think he'd ever even *know* about them. I certainly wouldn't have reached out if I'd been in my right mind.

I knew I'd inherited a few regrettable traits from him, but I've never figured out exactly what's wrong with my dad. Persecution complex? Delusions of grandeur? He claims that at one point he had a high-level security clearance with the Department of Defense. What would happen if I hooked him up to a lie detector with a gun to his head? Would he admit that he knew he didn't have a chance of making it in Hollywood? Would he admit to being a shitty father?

One thing that watching my father had taught me is that there is a real, and very important, distinction between sanity and lucidity. In my time at Bellevue and Good Shepherd, I'd lost both. My father, on the other hand, was arguably lucid—he spoke in sentences that made rough sense to strangers, he loosely understood cause and effect, and he was generally on the same page as everyone else regarding the properties of the physical world. But could you say that this man was "sane"?

It looked like he was trying to put on a concerned fatherly face, but I couldn't entertain the charade of "supportive parent" from him anymore. We snorted coke together until 8 a.m. the morning of my college Honor Society induction ceremony, for Christ's sake.

I broke. "So, what have you been up to?"

"Eh. You know…"

Please don't say pulling your head out of your ass.

"I'm getting my head out of my ass."

"Yeah, that's good."

"Got a few projects going."

"Oh yeah?"

"Yeah, tell me what you think of this. You know the album *Born to Run*?"

"The Boss? Yeah."

"That album…as a musical!"

Fuck me. "Yeah?"

"Yeah. You do it as a musical. Whatta you think?"

"Hm. Yeah, I guess it could be. Do you know anyone who does Broadway-type shows?"

"It would be more off-Broadway."

"Do you know anyone who does *off*-Broadway-type shows?"

"No. You could figure that out, though."

"Well, I'd say you might have trouble getting the rights."

"That's step one. Figure out who owns the rights."

"I think it's Bruce Springsteen." He laughed fairly hard, like I was being sarcastic. "But, yeah, if you can get the rights to *Born to Run*, I could see it as a musical."

"But what *I* want to know," he said with gusto, "is what is going on with *you*."

I told him that I'd just gotten out of the psych ward. That I have a pretty serious case of the bipolar. And that I was coming off a hard-core psychotic break. That's what was going on with me.

"I'm not sure I believe in bipolar disorder. What is bipolar anyway? It's a label we've made up."

"Yeah." He was right, to the extent that all words are labels we've made up — like "ball" or "car" or "cancer." But if words have meaning, I have bipolar disorder.

"So talk to me about this," he said.

"Mack..."

"Dad. I am your father."

"Honestly, no offense, but I think our relationship is what many therapists might call *estranged*. I don't know what you are hoping to accomplish here."

"I am trying to accomplish nothing. I want to understand. I seek understanding. This is what I seek." Sometimes he talks like this. I don't know how to describe his inflection other than *biblical*. "We don't know what the universe has in store for us," he continued.

"I can agree with that."

"We are not estranged either. We are here."

"Mack..."

"Dad."

"Okay," I said. "*Dad*. Historically, seeing you is hard. It brings up difficult emotions. I don't feel like confiding in you about this, and I hope you can respect that."

He looked a little hurt, which was fair.

"Fine. I can't make you do shit. No one ever could." It was obvious he thought I was being a petulant teen. I couldn't give him what he wanted, though.

We left it there and finished the meal in silence. He dropped me back off at the house and that was the last I saw of him for six years. I don't know what his intent was in visiting, but it did make an impact. I was twenty-eight, the same age he was when he moved to California. I'd been running my whole life from what Mack represents to me as a human being. It's no coincidence I ended up on the

East Coast. Law school, too, was a stand against Mack's Peter Pan life-style. Instant legitimate adulthood—that's what an LSAT score and $200,000 in loans buys you. You become "the lawyer in the family." It was proof that I wasn't a big damn joke. But all of a sudden, in spite of everything I'd worked for, I couldn't shake the fear that I was on the verge of becoming one.

To call the Bird a teacher would be like saying Obama was a civil servant. She is the lone teacher at the Urban League Learning Center. Her students are all high school dropouts. Many of them only attend classes to comply with probation. If I were a PD in Wichita, we'd know quite a few of the same people. Some I'd meet first; others I'd get after the Bird. For years now I've known she does the Lord's work, but I always have a renewed appreciation when I get to see her in action. Plus, she likes it when I drop by. The day after lunch with Mack, I did.

I surveyed her desk: a picture of Alexa in cap and gown at her vet school graduation, one of me standing in the East Village, and one of Adam in his high school cap and gown. I pointed out to her that she had a minor First Amendment violation in the form of a black Jesus calendar hanging over her desk.

"Boy, I am not here to argue logic or religion with you. I am here to graduate Coley Cole. Isn't that right, Coley Cole? You ready to do $y = mx + b$?"

"Whenever you ready," Coley Cole said.

"Do your thing," I told her.

I knew about Nacole "Coley Cole." She started coming to the Learning Center when she was twenty-eight years old. She had zero high school credits when she first started working with the Bird. Eight years later, they were still grinding toward her diploma.

Coley's mom left on her fourteenth birthday—she told her daughter she was going out to get a birthday cake and never came back. Even before that day, Nacole rarely lived with her mom for continuous stretches. Her home situation had been a series of foster homes and temporary stays with aunts and uncles in houses that were already four to seven people above capacity. She was never a welcome guest—food was already too scarce and she was just another mouth to feed. When she was nine, her thirteen-year-old cousin woke her up by smashing a dirty diaper in her face. Other cousins and uncles sexually abused her, and the foster system wasn't any better. Under the state's guardianship, she was sent to foster homes in western Kansas a handful of times, but she always left and walked back to Wichita. She'd be on the street or back to a different cousin's house, hoping—but not expecting—that each new arrangement might not be as bad as the last. The food situation was the lone consistency: there was never enough, and it was every man for himself.

While the Bird helped Coley Cole calculate the slope of a line—"It's $y = mx + b$. You know that, 'cause I told you that. There's your mx, now where's his brother b?"—three other students gathered around her, all working on different lessons. Maurice was trying to remember the principal interest rate equation: (i)nterest $= (p)$rincipal $\times (r)$ate / (t)ime. "You know prt. I equals p times r over t."

"What's the r stand for again?" Maurice asked.

"Not 'rich,' not for you," the Bird said, "not unless you can remember that it's 'rate'!"

The Bird has an avian-like ability to crane her neck around 270 degrees and keep a watch on all the other students under her tutelage without losing focus on the handful she is helping at any given time.

"Ms. Cindy, can I take a smoke break?"

"I know a smoke break takes seven minutes. But I'm nice. I'ma give you nine."

"You cool, Ms. Cindy."

"I'm cooler than cool. I'm cooler than a polar bear's toenails." Lines from an OutKast song. She memorizes a popular rap song or two at the beginning of every school year to keep in her back pocket and deploy as necessary.

"Smoke a Kool 100 for me. Or a Black and Mild."

She's at her best when students think they're in trouble — a common offense being looking up something inappropriate on the internet. The Bird can spot the offender even while spitting out quadratic equations, blessing smoke breaks, and letting brothers know they won't be rich if they can't remember that the *r* in prt stands for "rate." Wichita Unified School District 259 has wisely blocked access to all porn sites, but the Victoria's Secret website managed to squeak through the firewall. The Bird sauntered up to Marcus, a frequent offender, and sat down next to him. He tried to close the window on the sly, but the Bird made him open it back up.

"What part of the curriculum is this?"

Marcus said that he tried to look up "Christmas" and this is what happened.

The Bird asked him if he knew what "festive" and "garland" meant. She asked him if he knew what *Feliz Navidad* meant.

Marcus didn't know. "Sorry," he said.

"It's okay, I know it didn't have anything to do with those gorgeous women on the screen, because you don't care about that. You only care about the holidays and Christmas."

Students trickle in throughout the day at irregular intervals, some wearing ankle bracelets. She greets all of them individually and gets them clocked in and going on the computer. If a brother is wearing a pair of brand-new size 14 Jordans, she lets him know that she notices: the Bird will walk up to him, put her little size 5½ next to his skis, and ask, "Can I borrow those shoes this weekend?" One such brother told her "Ms. C-Mac, you blacker than black." His friend pointed to a picture of Terry on her desk and said, "Shit, she's black by injection."

She keeps a cache of personal hygiene products in her closet and doles them out as necessary. Her strategy there is to pull aside the *friend* of the student in need of soap or toothpaste or deodorant and hand them a goody bag. "Coley Cole, my friend works at Walgreens and I got all these free samples. Take 'em if you want, just share them, okay?" She doesn't take a lunch break, but she packs a lunch big enough to feed three men and complains of being too full. If she wants to make sure that some food makes its way to a mother she knows is having trouble feeding her kids, she hands them a sack of leftovers and says, "Can you take this home? I hate for it to go to waste. I don't have anyone at home to give it to." If they're really hard up, she gives them a Dillon's gift card wrapped in a note.

When young men walk in with hats on, she says, "Why are you doing that to me?"

"What?"

"Why are you denying me the opportunity to see your beautiful head?" If they have a good relationship, she changes it to "We know you have a big head. You can't hide it under that hat." Likewise, if a student she knows well summons her from across the room, she says, "Oh, sweetheart, I'm so sorry both of your legs are broken. Let me walk over there to you with my two perfectly good legs," then acts like she is too old to make it across the room while she drags one leg behind her. "I'm coming. Stay there." If she suspects a student won't return the next day, she says, "If you hear a loud explosion tomorrow morning, it's my heart breaking from across town."

There are two other facilities in Wichita that provide similar services—both have more teachers, more money, and more resources—and she logs more credit hours per year than both combined. She writes grants to get funding for bus fare. She brings in guest speakers—nurses, firefighters, pastors, a cop nicknamed "the white cop" by a seventy-year-old African American grandmother who is a few credits shy of graduating. The white cop is a popular speaker; he talks about community policing and tensions between law enforcement and black communities and doesn't shy away from questions.

It's been alleged that from time to time she's allowed a student to write a letter to an incarcerated family member instead of analyzing Mark Twain's *Last Words of Great Men*. "I don't love Mark Twain either," she's been accused of saying. "Make sure to tell your cousin that you are in school and doing well and that you're going to graduate."

At the end of the day she says, "Come back tomorrow. We open at eight, but I'll be here at seven. You can call me after five a.m. and before ten p.m. I hope I have convinced you that hanging out with me is more fun than sitting on the couch and waiting for your probation officer to come by. If it was hard, congratulate yourself on doing something brave today." And she always singles out the most frustrated student leaving the classroom at the end of the day. "You better watch out, Deshawn. You're going to graduate if you keep hangin' out with me."

"You a G, Ms. Cindy."

"I put the *O* in OG."

CHAPTER 20

I WAS BACK IN New York ten days after my discharge from Osawatomie. I just couldn't stomach a prolonged stay in Wichita and thought that, if I kept moving and dove back into my healthy pre-cornfield routine, I'd be able to move on from this experience more quickly. Take the punch and get up, go back to work, check in with Singh regularly—it seemed like a better recovery plan than the garage. There was rebuilding to be done for sure and depression felt imminent, but at least I hadn't lost my apartment this time; the Bird had made sure to get a rent check over to my roommates, kept me current on my bills, and stayed in touch with my supervisors at work.

I hadn't spoken to Jonas since the cornfield. I was afraid that our relationship had been irrevocably altered. I hoped it wasn't, but I needed to know for sure. In his circle, I had always been the stand-up with the screw loose. He was there when I dealt with a heckler by stripping down to my skimpy briefs, and when I did an entire set as an Olde Tyme baseball player riffing on my good friend Mark Twain, staying in character hours after getting offstage. Jonas knew I was crazy in the crazy-son-of-a-bitch sense, and he liked being friends with that crazy guy. But now he also knew I was just flat-out, literally crazy—the kind most people want to avoid.

I texted him the second night I was back in the city.

Pint tonight?

I'd eat.

K. San Marzano in an hour?

Sounds good.

I spotted his slow, wide-legged strut from a block away as I waited outside the restaurant and smoked a cigarette. He was wearing a beanie and his thick-heeled black boots that turn his five feet nine inches into five feet ten inches. We hugged when he got there and he held it a little longer than usual. "What's up, man? Good to see you! You look good!"

The waiter asked us if we wanted a drink. I thought I saw Jonas raise an eyebrow as I ordered.

"Yeah, fuck it. Me too." Jonas ordered a beer. "Fuck it, you can drink, right?"

"Yeah."

"It's good to see you, man."

"You too."

Perfectly cordial but definitely a bit stilted. I didn't know how we were going to kick this chat off, but luckily Jonas cut right to it. "So I got some shit to tell you. I just want to talk and I want you to listen. I just want to get this off my chest."

"Okay."

"I was pretty conflicted about what to do after all that shit went down. And I decided I have three options: One, I could have nothing to do with you at all. Quit hanging out with you. Cut you out of my life. Two, I could just go business as usual—keep hanging out with you, let you do whatever the fuck you want, smoke weed, get fucked-up, run around with you and chase women, all the same shit. Or, three, I could stay friends with you but alter my behavior around you and the way I handle you. And I decided, ultimately, on three."

"Huh. Okay," I said. *The way you handle me?*

"I was going to cut you off. When I came back from Wichita, I told my brother that I'm done. I'm done with that kid. I'm never fucking hanging out with him again."

"Okay."

"Just let me finish."

I waved both hands in a circular *Proceed* motion.

"Thank you. So I think I would have been well within my rights to cut you off. But I have some distance now, and I'm going to keep you in my life…"

I couldn't fully stifle an audible breath through the nose, inflating my chest a bit — the full-body version of an eye roll.

"But I'm not going to be an enabler anymore. I decided I will no longer enable you. I am not going to blow trees with you. I am not going to party late as fuck with you. I will never, never smoke weed with you again."

"Okay. Not a problem because I don't plan on smoking weed again."

"You don't know. You can't know that. You don't know what's wrong with you. You might be schizophrenic."

"I'm not."

"Your uncle was."

Pain was turning to anger. I was hearing *Congratulations. I am still going to be your friend.*

"You put me through a very fucked-up situation. You got us lost in a cornfield. It was cold as fuck. You were running around naked. You were…"

I got that few people want to chase their psychotic naked friend through permafrost in a cornfield in the dead of a Kansas winter. I got that it was scary. I got that it was an inconvenience. I even got that it might be a friendship deal breaker. But man did it hurt.

"And so that's what I'm going to do. I'm going to remain friends with you, but I don't want to travel with you. I don't want to take a road trip with you. My buddy and I are driving to the Outer Banks this weekend, and we're going to be blowing trees, and it's just something I would *never* invite you to anymore. I won't enable…I'm ready to hear what you have to say."

I couldn't look up. "Well, I don't really know what there is to say…"

"Come on. You always have something to say."

It was tempting to just leave. I'd never been read Terms and Conditions by a friend before. "Well," I started, "I guess if you want full, raw honesty…"

"When do we give each other anything else?"

"Right. So truth being—what you're saying fucking hurts. It hurts bad. I could cry if I let myself. And, honestly, I think it's fucked-up."

"Oh, come on, dude. You'd have done the exact same shit."

"No, I wouldn't. Not with you, not with any of my good friends."

"You don't know that. You weren't in my position."

"I do know. I wouldn't bail on you because you were sick. If you were sick, I'd visit you in the hospital."

"You can't know."

"I can fucking know and I do fucking know." The tears were just behind my eyeballs. "And I'm sorry, but I don't really see you as such a huge victim in all of this. What did you go through, really? You had a crazy fucking night—you were scared? You had to drive me to a fire station? You think that's how I wanted to spend my January? In a psych ward?"

"I was in Wichita, Kansas, by myself, for a fucking week. Didn't have shit to do but go to the Y and eat at the Hometown Buffet."

"That sounds like a pretty boring, shitty week, man. Sorry you had to go through that." We finished eating in silence. I was fighting the impulse to just throw down a twenty and say "See you at work. I don't need this."

But I did need him. I needed all the help I could get. His friendship had been huge in getting me through the last bout of depression. Now I was staring down that same dragon, wondering if it was even slayable.

We paid and left, the silence between us still dense. "Quick walk?" I asked.

"Yeah, we can do that."

We headed north to the East Village and by force of habit both stopped in front of one of our haunts. Inside he bought us two beers and we sipped in silence, until Jonas finally piped up. "Listen, man, I'm sorry. I didn't mean to hurt your feelings; I don't want to fight with you. I love you, man."

"I love you too."

I felt like I understood all the stories I'd heard about prison inmates having trouble adjusting after their release. The rhythms of Osawatomie followed me back to New York: I'd spend the first two hours of each day pacing the apartment, mimicking my daily routine at the hospital. I was used to watching my back, waiting for the next fight to break out, the next screaming maniac forced into isolation. *Eyes up, back against the wall, know your exits.* I'd pace without knowing it and then coach myself into embracing normal life: *You don't have to do this. You are allowed to sit down. You don't have to ask permission to watch TV. You can eat whatever you want for lunch. You can take a shower.* But I had developed a muscle memory for the aimless pacing and felt lost without someone telling me when to eat, when to shower, when to go to bed.

I'd also read enough about soldiers returning from Iraq with post-traumatic stress disorder to know that I had some form of it. My apartment left me feeling boxed in. I'd try to build up the courage to step outside, but the world out there seemed too chaotic to brave. I'd get excited that I was allowed to walk around my neighborhood, go wherever I wanted to go, but I felt tethered to my apartment as if I were attached by a cord that stretched only three blocks. Any farther and I felt like I had swum too far out to sea. My instinct said, *RUN! YOU'RE FREE!* but I was afraid to cross the street. The fear of catching a beatdown from a psychotic Gregory was replaced by the risk of getting hit by a car; the cacophony of the ward, by Manhattan's almost visible soundtrack.

Returning to work after my second psychotic break was in some ways harder than the first. I was embarrassed the first time. Now it felt like I'd been given a mulligan and wasted it. One psych ward, fine — we've all been there. But two? Two felt like a permanent rubber stamp that I was a certified fuckup. A pattern had been established: Every year, between the fall and winter, McDermott goes a little crazy and we have to lock him away for a while. Then he takes a big ol' long vacation and we see him again and he acts like nothing is wrong. Then he represents *our* crazy people — all the while, we know it's only a matter of time before he is off the rails again and we're here to clean up his mess.

I tried to do the same thing I'd done after my first leave: be on time, look professional, and cover cases when asked. The surest way to minimize embarrassment at the office and avoid sliding into another crippling depression seemed to be to throw myself back into work. Which is how I ended up conducting a cross-examination of the queen of France.

Debrah Turley was arrested for assault and she couldn't make the $500 bail. The tax on those too poor to make bail is paid in jail time. Two defendants, separated by $500 in net worth, charged with the same crime and with similar criminal records, could easily end up serving widely disparate jail sentences. If only she could have made bail, we'd have gotten her a non-jail sentence.

This situation plays out hundreds of times each day. But what made Ms. Turley's case memorable was that the alleged victim, her ex-girlfriend, was batshit, in the throes of psychosis, crazy.

In New York, it's legal to record any conversation as long as one party consents. That means, if I want to call a hostile witness and tape it, I can. This can be incredibly useful come cross-examination time, so I called Ms. Turley's ex, and for forty-five minutes she unwound her fantastic autobiography for me. She hailed from a long line of both French and English royalty—her grandfather was the king of France, and she was in line to become the queen—so her family was worth hundreds of millions of dollars and the CIA was following her per Obama's orders. Of course she was a Mason too, and she knew that I was one as well because she'd seen me "do some of the signs and signals in court. You adjusted your glasses, you were rubbing your eyes, running your hands through your hair, messing with your tie."

I usually felt nothing but contempt for adverse witnesses—a convenient attitude since the only purpose of our conversations was to gather ammunition to crucify them on the stand. But I was overwhelmed with compassion for Debrah's girlfriend, my opponent. She reminded me of so many lost souls I'd met at Bellevue. Who was going to help her put reality back together? How was she even going to feed herself? Here I was preparing to humiliate this woman, who had no idea I was her adversary, based on information I had gathered without her knowledge and at her most vulnerable point. If it weren't for the Bird, it could have been me on the other end of the line, claiming to be the duke of Wichita or, perhaps, a famous comedian.

But what could I do for her, or others like her? I could barely even help my client. I was way behind the curve as an attorney. I'd had two trials and won them both and felt confident in the courtroom, but I knew I was ignorant far too often on case law and criminal procedure. I wanted to start all over, go back to day one of misdemeanor training and pay attention this time. Instead of being cocky and acting like *I got this* all the time, admit that I knew nothing and soak it all in. But there was no time to reset. The NYPD kept beating and arresting the homeless, the helpless, the sick, and the poor. My phone didn't quit ringing off the hook. My only choice was to be confident in what I did know while trying to play catch-up where I could. But I wished I could do more.

CHAPTER 21

CHICO BORJA WAS THE only reason I'd come in to the office that day. I tossed Shaqon Barnett, Tamir Gray, and Abayomi Osu on the floor and opened Chico's file. On its merits, his case was not that serious: a simple assault charge stemming from an incident with his boyfriend. He had a good self-defense case and neither party suffered any physical injuries. But the top of his file was stamped ICE HOLD—Immigration and Customs Enforcement—a big problem.

The ICE hold meant that even if the judge was willing to release him, the Department of Corrections would still detain him until ICE picked him up. Chico's only prayer was for me to get his case dismissed outright. NY DOC won't hold you—even with an ICE hold—if your case is closed.

That was Chico's first problem but not nearly the most critical. Underneath the ICE stamp, I'd scribbled *730 issues, see inside flap*. When I'd met Chico in jail a few days earlier, his first words to me were "Mister, you have to get me out of here. I'm bipolar. I haven't had my medicine. I need my medicine." Breaking the news to a client that he's not going home is routine, but there was such fear in his eyes. He was shaking, and he was clearly confused. "Why, why can't I go home, mister?"

"You see this stamp?" I told him. "That means that no matter what the judge decides, he can't let you go. It's not even up to him. This is Immigration, *la migra*."

He was in the soup and he was in the soup good. We had a Spanish translator in the cell with us, but Chico's English was more than adequate. I asked the translator to leave. Even though I was Chico's advocate, I still needed to gain his trust. Having *two* people on the other side of the bars means *two* people the client must trust.

"They won't let you go because, technically, you're illegal."

"But I need my medicine! I didn't do nothing!"

"Right. But they are *accusing* you of doing something, so they can hold you. It's not even about if you're guilty or not at this point."

"But ask my boyfriend. He attacked me. I had a bat because I was scared. He's big. He was drunk."

"How big?"

"Like this much taller." He moved his hands apart six inches. "And he heavy. He strong."

Chico was probably five foot four and 160 pounds. I jotted down his version of the story; we still had to begin preparing his defense, but I feared the ICE hold rendered a lot of what he was saying irrelevant. Still, I needed him to know I cared and that he could trust me. Telling him *Don't worry, it doesn't matter, you're fucked anyway* probably wouldn't work.

"I need my medicine, mister."

"What do you take?"

"Risperdal, Depakote, Seroquel, some other stuff. I don't know; a lady helps me."

"I'll tell the judge you need medical attention. They'll give you meds in jail."

"Please, I can't go to the jail. I have to go home!"

Chico started crying. I could only partially imagine the hell that awaited him — BP1, off his meds for several days, probably getting deported, headed to the loudest, scariest place in the entire country, and desperately needing sleep to stay sane. And that was only Chico's second problem.

"I have the virus."

"HIV?"

"AIDS."

Jesus fucking Christ.

"Are you on meds for that?"

"Yes." He rattled off his cocktail, and I noted it in his file, right under UNDOCUMENTED, HONDURAS.

"I'll tell the judge, but I am going to ask to go to the bench so I don't have to announce it in open court, okay?"

"Please. Please. I have to get out of here. I need medicine."

"I can't get you out of here."

He put his head in his hands and continued to cry.

"Don't cry. You don't want to cry in here. I'm going to do everything I can for you; I just can't solve this right now. It's going to take time."

"Please." He kept crying.

"It's not a matter of *please*. If I could do anything right now, I would. I just can't. Stop crying, all right?"

I waited until he wiped his eyes before leaving the interview booth.

"If you're going to cry more, stay in the booth until you're sure you're done, okay?"

He nodded, head still in hands. "I can't go back to Honduras."

"Why?"

"I'm gay! They'll kill me!"

That actually might help him in an immigration proceeding. We could argue political asylum.

The next day, I went to see Chico again at Brooklyn House of Detention as soon as I had an opening in my schedule. It was appalling to see this sweet, scared man in a jailhouse beige jumpsuit. His stories of past abuse rang true. I believed that he was terrified of his boyfriend, that he had no intention of hurting him, that he just didn't want to get killed himself. How could a supposedly civilized nation expose him to a potential death sentence in his homeland as the result of a domestic dispute that he most likely didn't instigate and wanted no part of? Because that's what we were doing. I Googled "gay+human+rights+violations+Honduras." He wasn't exaggerating the threat to homosexuals in Honduras. I found plenty of research documenting hate crimes and murders against gay and transgendered Hondurans. In the U.S., he had a care team and access to medical treatment at a local clinic. No way he'd have the same back home.

Chico looked better, somehow — more lucid, less panicked — when I visited him. He was getting meds and he seemed psychologically stable. I told him I had an immigration lawyer on his case, and we were assembling the best case we could to keep him in the country. I touched base with his social worker and encouraged her to get letters together from anyone who'd be willing to vouch for Chico. We went through his family history and connections to the U.S. In a deportation hearing, it helps if the defendant has been in the country a long time or has American-born children or family.

With as many clients as I had, it could be difficult to put a face to a name in between court appearances. They became a charge and a docket number until I saw them again in court. That wasn't a problem with Chico — the abject terror in his eyes was stuck in my mind like a splinter as I thumbed through his file. I may have managed, barely, to avoid going through the system in the middle of a mental health crisis, but Chico and I weren't that different. The fear consuming him on his way to the detention center was no less severe than what I would have felt in the same situation. Incarceration was not part of his life's routine — this was his first brush with the absurdity and indifference of the system. AIDS, bipolar, abused, persecuted for your sexuality? You are not special. Against the wall, spread your butt cheeks.

My devotion to Chico's case was wearing me out. I'd been going at it for a week nonstop; I was so tired that I wanted to collapse and yet so full of anxious energy that I wanted to drop down for fifty push-ups at least ten times a day. I spoke to every immigration lawyer in my office and tried to educate myself on the deportation process. I wanted to know his odds, even if those odds were: fucked. The answers I got from Immigration were complex and varied, but all led to the same conclusion: fucked.

Immigration policy is, in some ways, more draconian than the criminal justice system. I'd already done "enough" to address the immigration issue, meaning my ass was covered as far as due diligence was concerned. I'd prepared a far more detailed dossier to kick upstairs to the immigration unit than was required, but how much was really enough when Chico might die? Was the sleep deprivation worth the risk of a psychotic break of my own? What if I could only nominally increase his chances of release? And what about my other clients, whose files were stacked up on the floor? Abayomi Osu wanted to be the first member of her first-generation Nigerian family to go to college. If we didn't get her case dismissed, financial aid was out. And sometimes it's better to fold 'em in ICE cases like Chico's: plead guilty and let ICE do their worst. Honduras might not be where Chico wanted to end up, but it's a better destination than an immigration detention center and *then* Honduras. I feared we were delaying the inevitable.

No matter what, Chico had no hope of getting out any time soon. And I certainly couldn't do anything for him if I ended up in the hospital. Panic at nighttime is one thing, but it was 10:20 a.m. and I was on day two of no sleep when I wrapped up my latest jail conference with Chico. Anxiety was starting to devour me. I couldn't endure this for another twelve hours. I needed to shift my concern for Chico to concern for myself. *Walk away. For everyone's sake,* I thought, *you need to walk away.* Then I braced for the next wave of internal chatter: *You can save Chico's life. How can you possibly even think about leaving?* Fight or flight was battering me around. Leaving the office that night, I finally settled on flight, silently promising Chico that I wouldn't take a minute longer than necessary to get my own mental state back in order before returning. The plan was to go home, take a Risperdal, and pass out by 8 p.m.

Just then my phone buzzed with a text from my roommate: We've got bedbugs. What time can you be home?

Panic. New Yorkers lose their apartments to these things. Exterminators cost thousands of dollars and many landlords try to dick tenants into paying for it. Instead of popping a Risperdal and falling asleep, now I had to deal with these little fuckers.

The mood was somber when I got home: devastation coupled with suspicion. One of us had brought the bedbugs into the apartment, and instinctually, all three of us were wondering who to pin the blame on. Ryan, who traveled frequently and stayed in a different—though no doubt fancy—hotel every weekend? Preston, who ate beef stew from a can every night? For some reason, that little tidbit seemed highly indicative of guilt. Or what about me, the public defender who hugged a homeless guy every other day?

"So what's the move?" I said, forcing a can-do tone, trying to ignore the fear of what would almost certainly happen if I didn't get to sleep within the next few hours.

Beef Stew explained that we had to bag our shit, dry-clean it all, vacuum every corner of the apartment, and cook all of our shoes along with anything else the bugs could possibly hide in.

"What can they hide in?"

"Everything."

I threw away every nonessential piece of clothing I owned. I couldn't afford to dry-clean all that shit. My rule was, if I hadn't worn something in the last month, it was gone. My panic fed on itself as twenty minutes turned into three hours. *Fifteen more minutes. Another half hour. Fuck, it's almost midnight. We aren't close to done.* Every minute that passed felt like a minute closer to the psych ward.

When you have bedbugs, you are supposed to sleep with as little skin exposed as possible. I put on an old pair of track sweatpants and tucked them into a pair of soccer socks. I tucked a long-sleeve T-shirt into my underwear. I even put socks on my hands for a minute before determining it to be utterly ridiculous. By that point I didn't care if the bedbugs ate me alive and left only my bones; I just needed sleep before it was too late. I knew I needed to take Risperdal, but it had gotten so late that I worried it would knock me out too hard and I wouldn't wake up for work in the morning. *Maybe I'm tired enough I don't need it.* I held the tiny orange pill in my hand and went back and forth for ten minutes.

I didn't take it. Big mistake.

CHAPTER 22

INSOMNIAC ENERGY SURGED THROUGH me all night. Each glance at the clock spawned a new wave of anxiety. The anxiety led to anxiety over the fact that my anxiety was going to prevent me from falling asleep. I never quit deliberating whether or not to take the Risperdal, but as sleepless minutes turned into sleepless hours, the risk of taking it and then not being able to wake up increased. When I did sleep, I dreamed that the bugs were crawling on me.

The next morning, once I finally convinced myself to leave my apartment, I could feel my grasp on reality loosening as I walked to the F train. I focused on my normal routine: walk the five blocks down Rivington to Essex, stop at the Essex market to get a $2 coffee from Porto Rico, wait for the train while I listen to the elderly Chinese man play the erhu, wish that the elderly Chinese man would quit playing the erhu. The routine was comfortable. One foot in front of the other, and soon I'd accomplished steps one through three of getting through my day—leave, coffee, train. *If you just stay slow and steady, deliberate and calm, you can make it through the day.*

As the F made its way under the East River into Brooklyn, the concept of sleep began to feel like a theoretical need more than a natural human function. Cognitively, I knew I needed it, but it felt as if my body had forgotten how to shut down. We pulled into the York Street station in Brooklyn; only one more stop until I'd have to get off the train and go play lawyer. I shut my eyes and tried to take deep breaths. *You've done this a thousand times. You can do it again.* My eyes felt like they'd retreated into the back of my skull and were floating around inside my head.

I clutched my backpack to my chest—hugging it for comfort, really—and fantasized about the moment when I would be able to try and sleep again. *I should just let myself conk out and ride this train to Coney Island and back.* I knew I'd be okay if I could just do that—give myself two hours of sleep.

"Jay Street Metrotech. Next stop Bergen Street. Stand clear of the closing doors!"

Here we go. *Focus on the familiar.*

I took the stairs up the platform two at a time. I was an object in motion and I needed to stay in motion. I passed the homeless guy who sits on a milk crate at the top of the F platform at Jay Street every day. He had a Duane Reade bag full of Duane Reade bags. Whether it was August or February, he always wore the same heavy winter coat and smoked Newports.

Focus on the familiar.

The first thing I saw when I entered my office was a note on my chair: *See me when you get in.*

Godfuckingdammit.

It was from Barry. I started thinking of reasons I couldn't cover whatever case it was he needed me to cover. My desk was in complete squalor. *What the fuck is wrong with me?* The stacks of files, piles of missing discovery, discarded depositions, unfiled recordings of 911 calls, and mosaics of sticky notes plastered to my phone, keyboard, and computer monitor weren't a reflection of a young devoted go-getter who'd just been working too darn hard. I couldn't even remember what message corresponded to what case on more than half the stickies. **Call back 718-212-8217.* Did the star mean it was important? Important enough to not write down whether it was a client, a witness, a social worker, a DA, a detective, or an investigator?

Public defenders always have ten or twenty balls in the air. Organization is a virtue, but files get left open when the phone rings and you're forced to switch gears to talk to a DA about a different case than the three you already have open. Or a client stops in, unannounced and with no appointment. Sometimes the only thing you can do is toss everything on the floor and pull the most important case you're working on in the moment, trusting that you'll get to the rest when *they* become the most important. Triage.

And who's this darkening my doorway now? Mr. See Me When You Get In.

"Calendar says you're going to courtroom TP-5; can you cover a case for Alinari? She's out sick." He had no idea that this routine favor he was asking from me would be the last little nudge that sent me over the edge.

"Barry, I need a minute. I don't think I can."

"But you're going, right?"

"I don't know."

"What do you mean you don't know? You have…"

"Tamir Gray."

"Right, Tamir Gray. Is it not on?"

"No, it's on. I just…"

Barry clearly thought I was just being lazy. I scanned for the right words — calm, collected words that would explain my current state of mind — but I came up empty.

"Barry, I can't do this! I'm so fucked! I'm fucked! Fucked!" I started crying, then bawling, then hyperventilating. *What a fucking fraud. You can't do shit for anyone!* "Shut the door. Please, shut the fucking door, Barry."

Barry sighed. He hates putting out fires, and as supervisor of our unit, putting out fires was 90 percent of his job.

"First, calm down."

"I can't calm down! I'm going to have to take a leave of absence! I can't do this! I'm sorry, I'm sorry, I'm sorry!" I couldn't stop crying.

"Let's take this one step at a time. What do you have on today besides the TP-5?"

"I don't know. Two domestic violence cases and then a bunch of other cases everywhere else."

"Okay, can you write coverage notes?"

"I can't do shit. I can't think. I'm so tired I'm seeing colors."

"Okay, I'll write the notes."

"That's not the problem. This guy right here"—I held up Chico's file—"AIDS, gay, bipolar, illegal. He's going to get deported, and he's innocent."

Barry fidgeted with his wedding ring. "Hand me the file." He skimmed through my notes and the discovery material. Within about a minute, he seemed to have absorbed everything he needed to know about the case. "I had a supervisor back in the old days who used to say to me 'This building won't burn down if you're not here. It was here before you and it will be here after you.' We have a hundred twenty-five other capable lawyers here. You aren't the first person to come undone in this place and you *definitely* won't be the last either. I got Mr. Borja. Go."

Barry shut the door behind him and I picked up my phone and scrolled to DR. SINGH 911—his emergency line. Just seventy-two hours earlier I had thought I could literally, maybe, save a goddamn life. As things stood, I felt more like a helpless accomplice to murder.

"Hello, this is Dr. Singh."

I wasn't prepared for him to answer; I'd planned on leaving a message and collecting myself before he called me back.

"This is Zack McDermott." I was already crying again before I got "McDerm" out of my mouth.

"You don't sound good."

"I'm *not* good!" I grabbed my hoodie off my chair and buried my face in it to keep the other lawyers from hearing me sob. It probably didn't work.

"No, you don't sound good...not good at all." His voice was the very embodiment of serenity. Just as a man in a cell explaining to me why he'd been forced to "lay hands on her" had become entirely mundane to me, Dr. Singh was surely desensitized to the vast majority of calls he received from the panicked, deranged, and suicidal. News of this little incident wouldn't even make it to his dinner table. "You sound like you might need to go to the hospital."

"I'll go, but you can't let them hold me! You can't let them hold me!"

"I think you need to get in a cab. Go. Go now. I'll call Beth Israel and see if they can admit you — First Avenue and Sixteenth Street." He was silent on the issue of letting them hold me; of course it was a promise he couldn't make.

I walked halfway down the block, hopefully out of view and earshot of any other attorneys, and screamed into the wind. I surveyed the downtown Brooklyn foot traffic: old lawyers waddling to court like penguins, a horde of mostly young African American men headed in the same direction. McDonald's was packed, and the line at the Social Security Disability office that shares our building was already snaking around the corner. *Take a good look; you might not be outside again anytime soon.* I hailed a cab.

"Beth Israel, please."

He hit the gas pedal like he had a gunshot victim in the backseat.

"You don't have to drive fast," I said. "I'm in no hurry."

I called my mom as we headed over the Brooklyn Bridge into Manhattan. Even though she was at school, she picked up quickly. For three years now, she'd lived in fear of this exact call.

"What's up, Gorilla?"

I was still crying but no longer gasping. "I'm headed to the hospital."

"What's wrong?"

"I haven't slept for three nights. I'm having a panic attack. I'm afraid I'm going to be manic if I can't fall asleep. I couldn't sleep last night. I was going to take a Risperdal. But we have bedbugs."

"Oh no. That's not good."

"No."

"You know where you are? You don't think you're on TV?"

"No, not yet. I don't want to fucking go to the fucking hospital."

It was obvious she was now softly crying too. "I don't want you there either. But if you have to go, you have to go. You're doing the right thing."

"I'll call you when I can."

"You don't want me to stay on the phone with you?"

"No. I want to roll the window down and feel some air before they lock me up in there."

"Okay."

"I love you," I said.

"I love you too. You're a strong gorilla. Call me as soon as you can."

I counted in my head how many blocks we had left when we exited the bridge: Canal, Grand, Broome, Delancey, Houston, then First through Sixteenth, and that was it.

"You okay?" the cabdriver asked me.

"Yeah, just fucked-up. You can take your time. Really."

He gunned it again. I estimated I had, at best, seven more minutes.

"We are here," he announced in five. "No charge."

"It's okay." I began to pull out my credit card.

"No charge. You go."

CHAPTER 23

I SURRENDERED MY CLOTHES and changed into green scrubs—the uniform of the insane. It's a small indignity but unquestionably degrading, the beginning of the infantilizing loss of autonomy. On admission, I was tranq'd up with two milligrams Risperdal and two milligrams Ativan and placed in a small white room. To a sane person, the room would have looked perfectly serene. But this seemingly serene room pulsed and banged, the storm in my head radiating an almost kinetic output of angst.

"I need more Risperdal and Ativan," I told the attending nurse. "I can tell I am about to break. No question."

"What's that mean?"

"I just know. I can feel it. I just keep thinking about how fast my brain is. I'm terrified. I need to sleep."

"We'll call the doctor. Go lie down until then."

Over the next hour, as I lay in bed waiting for the doctor, the room grew increasingly menacing. I became terrified that the thick rectangular light cover would somehow come loose and fall on me, creating a bloody mess. I couldn't quit staring at it; it looked so unstable. *Why do we trust the construction of buildings and fixtures so blindly? Why are we not constantly terrified that the walls will come crashing down?* I was hanging on to that last grain of reason that told me these thoughts were irrational, that New York City has building codes, that

Sheetrock is a tried-and-true building material, that the screws and nuts and bolts were installed by certified union carpenters. But that was of little comfort. *Yeah, your train is headed off the rails. Wait for it — should happen any minute now.*

The doctor knocked and let himself into my room without waiting for an answer. "So you can't sleep yet?" he asked. "Not at all?"

"Nothing. No sleep. Can't sleep. And I'm getting bad."

"What do you mean?"

"Manic. Not psychotic yet, but I can feel it coming. The walls are moving."

"What do you mean, 'The walls are moving'?"

"The angles look all wrong, like it's not a parallelogram. It's askew."

"But you know they're fine, right?"

"Yeah, I'm sure they're fine. But they don't *look* fine to me. And I know *I'm* not fine."

"What else makes you think you're manic?"

"I can tell I'm starting to think I have better extrasensory perception than I know I should have. Like, I'm seeing things almost before they happen. But I *know* that I can't be."

"It seems you are anxious, but you still aren't struggling to separate perception from reality."

"That's accurate. I don't want it to start, though. You have to give me something else. I have to sleep."

He instructed the nurse to give me the max Risperdal dose. It was a relief to throw some more pharmaceuticals down the hatch, but it also felt like we'd just fired our last bullet. *Why isn't this shit working already?*

I was still awake an hour after the final dose. Then another hour. Then another. I tried repeating a mantra that made sense to me at the time: *If you're breathing, you aren't dead. If you're breathing, you can't die.*

I was trying to white-knuckle myself sane.

The same doctor came in to check on me the next morning. It must have been the end of his shift. "So how'd we do? Sleep?"

"No sleep." I was near tears.

"I'm disappointed to hear that. I'm afraid that we're going to have to move you."

"Not Bellevue. Please, you can't send me to Bellevue. I can't go to Bellevue."

"Not Bellevue. We're going to send you to Gracie Square. They have a bed for you. It's a private hospital."

I was strapped to a gurney and loaded up by two EMTs.

When it comes to loony bins, "private" does not necessarily mean "better." Gracie Square looked like a dystopian government facility where the patients are experimented on. There *weren't* old metal buckets catching water drops from rotting ceilings or live electric wires snaking along the ground, but it felt like someone would be along any minute to install them. I would have switched my lease over to Bellevue without a second thought.

The clientele was even worse. They were all angry—hateful, even. I needed a good cry, but not in the hall. I was still fresh meat.

I felt twenty sets of eyeballs on me while the *one* staff member on duty showed me around. It was on him to keep pace with thirty or forty severely mentally ill patients, and he was flailing. I saw him break up three fights in the first hour; he had to make a snap decision each time on who to tackle and restrain, and then hope the other person would voluntarily back off. It was unclear whether he went for the aggressor or the easier person to subdue; the latter seemed like a more prudent strategy. I bet the guy didn't make $40,000 a year. *What is the backup plan if someone incapacitates him? Inmates running the asylum?*

"What *is* this place?" the tiny young girl sitting next to me in the cafeteria asked me. Her face was beet red and splotchy like an old drunk in his fifties. Her nose seemed to be growing sideways. I imagined her breath didn't smell good, even after brushing. It looked like she'd been crying for days, and it was obvious she was terrified to be here.

"Psych ward."

"I don't know what the fuck I'm doing here."

"Well, if you need to be here…"

"I wanted rehab. I'm not crazy."

"So why here?"

"I don't know. I went to the hospital; I had my stomach pumped for the third time. My parents won't talk to me unless I go to rehab."

She lifted her legs so her feet rested on the cold metal bench, pulled her knees to her chest, and burrowed her head as far down as it would go. I could feel where Red was coming from. She didn't have that hard bark on her. Plus, she was tiny.

"Look," I told her, "get out of here. Whatever your problem is, this is not the solution."

"I just wanted help and they put me in this hellhole!"

"It is a hellhole. This is the worse one I've ever seen."

"I'm scared I'll get drunk. I'll leave and go get drunk. I *want* to be locked up somewhere. I'll drink otherwise. I know I'll drink."

"Know what I think? I think the longer you stay here, the greater the odds you are going to go get fucked-up when you leave. This isn't going to straighten you out. Call your dad, tell him you're sorry, tell him you'll sew your mouth shut, tell him anything. But you need to leave."

I was released four days later. The antipsychotics they gave me had pushed me into a semi-comatose state. Friends made visits I don't remember, but eventually the drugs knocked me out fully and I was able to string together two nights of good sleep.

It was unseasonably warm for February when I stepped back into the world. I decided I'd walk the seventy-eight blocks home from the hospital. I was dazed and relieved to be out, but I was also pissed. It was just over a year since I'd left Osawatomie. I was following the rules: making sure I slept enough, taking my meds every morning, and smoking zero pot. And yet, I was once again walking out of a psych ward. My mind had violated the pact.

I called Singh on my walk home to let him know I was out and to schedule a follow-up appointment. He asked me how I was doing. *Pissed. Annoyed. Embarrassed. Defeated.* I told him I didn't know what to do. That a yearly crisis of some magnitude seemed to be inevitable; that it's terrifying that one little ill-timed bedbug incident sends me straight to the ER. Basically, what the hell am I supposed to do, here?

"If there's one thing we know with you," Dr. Singh said, "it's that once an acute manic or psychotic episode starts, it becomes wildfire incredibly fast. And we missed it here. The Risperdal early keeps everything nice and wet. No fire."

The world was eating lunch and headed in every imaginable direction. It was reaffirming to be back in the gen pop, and my talk with Singh helped me begin to shed some of the antsiness brought on by my confinement. He was right: while it was hard to celebrate a small victory when the "victory" was four days in a psych ward, four days really was a victory of sorts, maybe even a huge one. I'd managed to avoid psychosis. No fire.

I found myself smirking at the BP. *You tagged me again, but you only landed a glancing blow. I'm figuring you out.*

CHAPTER 24

SHE WAS STANDING ON the sidewalk smoking a cigarette and laughing with her friend. *That girl is too beautiful to be here,* I thought. *And you probably have about five seconds to get your moxie up before another guy does.* She had a natural pout that kind of made her look like a French bulldog — adorable but a little grumpy.

Bumming a cigarette was my obvious entrée. But it was her friend who gave me the cigarette, leaving me with the task of keeping them both entertained while simultaneously making it clear that it wasn't her friend I was trying to talk to.

I could tell she was foreign by the way she gestured and held her cigarette like she couldn't be bothered. No fake smiles or exaggerated laughs. And once I got closer, the French accent. She introduced herself as "Michelle from Texas" and I pretended to believe her.

"Oh yeah? What part?"

"Da middle."

"Mmmm, the middle's nice."

It was late and I figured they were leaving, but her friend said we should all go inside and get another beer. "Where are your friends?" Michelle from Texas asked me.

"I was just trying to figure that out. Somewhere — they're here somewhere."

"You don't have any friends, do you?"

"That's what I'm starting to worry about."

An obnoxious future Wall Streeter did me a huge favor by over-aggressively flirting with Rachel, her friend. "You ever heard of NYU Stern? It's one of the best MBA programs in the country." While he ran down his CV for Rachel, I did my best animal impressions for Michelle from Texas: Gila monster, killer whale, camel, giraffe (very similar to camel), and bald eagle. She loved the story I told her about a client who was arrested for walking the Coney Island boardwalk with a boa constrictor wrapped around his neck; he claimed to be famous and said, "Been doing this for twenty years, man!"

She told me, "You're a bullshitter. King of da bullshit is what I would call dat." I liked being King of da Bullshit—couldn't ask for a better title. But then she said, "You should kiss Rachel so dat dis fucking idiot will go away."

"Me go away?"

"You seem like a good idiot. You can stay."

No way I was kissing Rachel. I had her laughing, and *this* idiot was staying. I left the bar with her number—I think I sealed the deal when I correctly guessed how to spell her real name. "A-U-R-E-L-I-E with an accent over the first *e*?"

"Thank God you don't make me play da monkey and ask me seventeen times how does it spell. Dat's why I have to be Michelle from Texas. Everybody plays da monkey." She asked me where I thought she was from.

I had no idea, so I guessed: "Not France."

Belgium.

Twenty minutes into my first date with Aurélie, I was making would-you-rather deals with the universe: *If you tell me right now that I have to marry this girl or never see her again, it's forever and it's not even close.* She said I sounded like a cowboy, that I must come from "*L'Amérique profonde.* Da real America." She called all insects "flies"—except butterflies, which she called "lullabees"—even the wasps that made her scream in terror. "It's a fly! I am scared of da flies!" She was so gorgeous I could barely swallow it. She had these little curls at the top of her hairline and she wore a thin red headband a few inches past her forehead. I figured that people had been telling her they loved her little angel hairs her whole life and wondered if she was self-conscious about them.

It had been four months since I'd walked home from Gracie Square. As far as psych ward hospitalizations go, it had been a relatively speedy rebuild. But could I have imagined on that mid-February walk that by Memorial Day I'd be sipping a beer in the sun closing out a first date to end all first dates? Nah, not really, and fucking A.

She proposed a beach day on City Island for our third date. Shit. With back hair thick enough to comb, this gorilla is more at home in a temperate climate. But it was a ninety-degree June afternoon and I couldn't think of a plausible reason to turn her down, so I resigned myself to lying on my back and keeping Aurélie in front of me at all times. Our collective ignorance of the Bronx really bailed me out—it's an island with no beach! We walked around for hours, her bummed that we couldn't find any sand, me secretly thrilled and saying, "Jesus, what kind of an island…?" like all I wanted for Christmas was a beach volleyball game. Instead, we passed the day people-watching and perusing gift shops that somehow stayed open peddling sterling-silver dreamcatcher earrings.

Aurélie and I spent an inordinate amount of time envisioning the woman who would happily receive this jewelry as a gift and pop them straight into her ears as soon as she opened the velvet cube. "Well, bless your heart! These are going to go so well with my amethyst." Her name is Tammy, there are quite a few aqua-colored knits in her wardrobe, and she wears her hair in what might be called an "inverted spiky bob." A few long, asymmetrical strands hang down the side of her face, the top of her head is a teased-out nest of controlled chaos.

Her stylist has trimmed it shorter down the back of her head to her neckline, which has been roughly squared off with electric clippers. No fewer than four earth-tone hues were used in her streaky highlights, but yellow is the dominant color, no doubt.

"It's like da—who is da guy dat's made of straw dat you put in da countryside?"

"Scarecrow."

"Yeah, like da scarecrow—because it's yellow like da straw, but it's all da colors of da fall, because da farmers dress da straw man to look like da leaves."

By midday I was pretty sure her dad was dead. I could tell she was having fun, but even as we expanded Tammy's bio over the course of the next few hours, there was a melancholy that tagged along behind her. Over beers at sunset, when I asked her what her parents did, I sort of knew what was coming.

"My mom is an accountant and my dad is dead."

"Sorry." That's all I said.

"I don't remember him." That's all she said.

I wondered how her experience of not having a father had differed from mine, if it hurt worse to have never known him than to have known him and then have him leave. Probably pros and cons to both.

Either way, the question didn't sink her mood. She was enraptured by the boats on the water. "I gotta get a boat, man. How do you get a boat?" she said. "Dese people on dese boats don't know how lucky dey are."

I made a mental note to get her a boat.

She spread her arms wide and asked me, "What do you call da, oh Jesus...all da...everywhere? All da blue?"

I had no idea what she was talking about. She was gesturing at the water and the heavens and the bar and the boats.

"With da white?" She didn't seem to have a clue what she was look-ing for. "White? Blue?"

"Smurf? I don't know."

"You kind of look like Papa Smurf with your *barbe*."

"Barb?"

"Beard. Big beard. Skee? What's da skee called? All da blue. It's easy…"

"Sky?" I guessed.

"Sky. I'm an idiot monkey."

I wondered if it would ever get old trying to understand each other. In the best way, I was suddenly feeling like I didn't have enough years left to live.

After the City Island jaunt, she basically moved in. I got the story of how her dad died: brain tumor when she was only a year old. After that, her grandparents lived with her and her mom. They slept upstairs on two twin beds pushed together to make one. She considered *Bon-Papa* her dad. He took her to feed the ducks and did all manner of absurd amateur science experiments with her. He loved to smoke *le pipe* and watch *le football* on their tiny TV.

She was nine years old when *Bon-Papa* died. She still can't stand the smell of eucalyptus because, when he was dying in the hospital, the nurses put eucalyptus in the humidifier in his room. Shortly after he passed, the doctor said it would be good for her to come into the room and say goodbye. She did, but even at that age, she knew he couldn't hear her. When people are gone, they're just gone — her mom had never told her any differently.

Then her mom got cancer. Aurélie was sure she'd die too and soon she'd be all alone — no *Bon-Papa*, no ducks, no Dad, no *Maman*.

We both smoked like hell; we drank a bottle of cheap champagne and smoked a pack of Marlboro Reds together almost every night that summer while we talked until bedtime. I talk too much, but I loved hearing her voice so I tried to make myself shut up so she'd talk more. I loved her accent — French with a little Kermit the Frog mixed in. We spent so much time together and her English was so new and impressionable that soon this little frog-voiced Belgian developed a rather salty vocabulary and picked up a slight Wichita drawl. When she'd tell her friends back home she was dating a guy from Kansas, the immediate response was usually "Is he a cowboy? Like *Walker, Texas Ranger*?" — apparently Chuck Norris is huge in Belgium. When she'd add that my name is Zack — not a name they have there — the follow-up became "Like *Saved by the Bell*?" "Yes, exactly like dat," she always said. "I tell dem you are a pretty blond high school cowboy."

On Saturday mornings she talked to her *Maman* in the loudest, fastest French I'd ever heard as she paced back and forth on my deck and burned through half a pack of cigarettes. When I'd ask her what they were fighting about, she'd say, "Nothing. She was just telling me dat Victor was rolling in his shit in da garden again and killed a bird and brought it into da house." That was usually the extent of the news from Belgium. Forty-five minutes yielded a dog report with a few crime statistics peppered in for good measure. She insisted that crime in Brussels was on a level that I failed to appreciate and that they rob old people there. She worried about her mom all the time. Worried she'd get robbed. Worried she'd get sick again. Worried she should be back in Belgium with her.

Like most have-not lovebirds in New York, our weekend dates defaulted to aimlessly walking around the city. It was on one of these epic walks that I had a dizzying and semi-disturbing realization: I had a grand Oedipal complex. We were walking by one of those $19 bottomless brunch places when Aurélie just went *in* on the clientele: "Drinking in da middle of da day. Brunch is not for drinking. Who are dese people, getting dressed up like dey are going to da discotheque for brunch? You aren't supposed to put on makeup to go eat da pancakes; you're supposed to be in your pajama. It's da girls dat lose dere shoes at night." I recognized this attitude immediately. I was dating a young, foreign, misanthropic granny.

* * *

I was afraid for her to know about my condition too soon. How do you explain to the woman you've fallen in love with that you have a little secret it's time to share, and then casually toss off that you've spent some portion of your life in a state of manic psychosis? *Hey, Aurélie, I think you're incredible and you're my new favorite person on the planet and, by the way, sometimes I'm psychotic."* "Bipolar," "psychotic," "insane" — it's still 100 percent okay to use these words as pejoratives; they are our go-to labels to describe dangerous people. I've never heard *anyone* be chastised or corrected for flippantly describing a person as "fucking crazy." There's a consensus in our society that the mentally unstable are to be avoided if at all possible. What would any well-intentioned friend advise her upon hearing that she was falling for a manic-depressive who in the recent past had involuntarily spent well over a month committed to four different psychiatric wards as a result of a disease for which there is no cure?

It helped that she'd told me about *Bon-Papa* and her dad's death and her mom's illness. I knew she understood trauma, and I had a pretty good read on her level of empathy and open-mindedness. I'd never seen someone throw a dirtier stank eye than when she witnessed a handful of people cover their noses when a car-clearing homeless man, reeking so strongly of piss and shit that I had to suppress my own gag reflex, boarded the train. She'd also become obsessed with prison documentaries and — after she learned about the prevalence of wrongful convictions, coercive interrogations, police brutality, and "lifestyle crimes," such as taking up two seats on the subway — took to hating the NYPD nearly as much as I do. "Da fucking pigs on da train harassing dis homeless guy who is just standing dere not bothering anybody," she'd begin. "It makes me sick. I want to just hit dem. And da stupid foreign tourists taking pictures with dem."

So I sensed she could handle heavy stuff, and even though we hadn't said it yet, I knew she loved me. There was no way to tiptoe around the subject, so one evening on my deck, halfway through our champagne and cigarettes, I just laid it all out there: the hospitalizations, the psychosis, the depression, the PTSD, and the permanence of it all. I explained that it's something I *have,* not something I *had.* I told her about my medication regimen and how, if I don't get enough sleep, I freak out that I'm going to have to go to the hospital again. I told her that I take pills every morning and that I'll have to for the rest of my life. I told her about just how terrifying the whole thing can be when I get too close to the ledge. Not just for me but for everyone around me. I told her about Gregory and Monk Monk, and Osawatomie, and Bellevue, and Gracie Square. About how the depression that follows the manic, like night follows day, put me on a lawn chair in my mother's garage for two months and put a six-pack down my throat nightly, and about how it had me listening intently to oncoming subway trains. About how it nearly ended my career as a lawyer and definitely ended my career in comedy. I told her about how bipolar disorder had very nearly fucking broken me and might yet still.

She teared up a little and held my hand. I teared up a little. It was the first time I'd ever told my story to someone who I needed to accept me. The moral of the story was clear: if you're with me, you're likely signing up to go through some shit.

"I don't care at all. It doesn't matter. Doesn't change anything. Nothing," she said. "I care because it happened to *you,* but I don't care dat you have dat. You're you." I was relieved by her reaction, but I was also aware that I couldn't take this as her final answer. *You're you.* How could she know what that meant when she hadn't seen all of me? When she hadn't seen my disease.

CHAPTER 25

THREE MONTHS LATER WE were standing in city hall waiting for a judge to approve our expedited marriage license and assign us an officiant to swear our sacred oath. We'd known each other for five months and seventeen days. It was a Thursday.

She went first to the kiosk where the bride and groom have to fill out their pedigree information, punching in "Aurélie" in the FIRST NAME field. Then, in the adjacent field, the screen asked for LAST NAME. She looked up at me. "Hagen, right?"

"Yeah, Hagen."

When they finally called McDermott-Hagen, we were ushered into Chapel 4. The officiant, a round man with a dark moustache and a heavy Brooklyn accent, was resplendent in a boxy khaki suit with a dress shirt the color of a secluded Caribbean bay and a tie the color of Sunkist. I asked him if he'd mind if I set up a camera.

Judging by the pace of the turnover in the courthouse chapels, it was his fiftieth ceremony of the day, and he was well into his opening remarks by the time I had the angle right. But what he lacked in patience he more than compensated for with a snake-handling, speaking-in-tongues level of secular fervor. "FROM THIS DAY, TO YOUR LAST, SHALL YE SWEAR OFF ALL OTHERS…BY THE POWER VESTED IN ME, BY THE GREEEEAAAT! STATE OF NEW YORK…" The man had stage presence. Aurélie and I practically had to stick our fists into our mouths to avoid full-on cracking up.

Rachel from the bar stood next to Aurélie, and two expats—Gaelle (BEL) and Benjamin (FRA)—rounded out the bridal party. Rachel and Gaelle cried; Benjamin very much needed to get back to work. I'd met each of them once.

On my side, Omar stood next to Ryan—two friends who had started as Craigslist roommates. Among all my friends, they probably understood my illness the best. Omar's father is BP1 and he doesn't take the best care of himself. Ryan's brother is schizophrenic; his whereabouts are unknown. Both had visited me at Gracie Square. Omar had brought me socks and underwear, and Ryan had given the Bird daily updates. I gave the best man nod to Jonas; he'd seen me shove my hand up my ass as he drove me out of a frozen cornfield. Safe to say he had a pretty good grasp of what my disease looked like.

The decision to get married had been made so quickly that there was no chance for the Bird to join. Besides, given the emergency flights and motel bills she'd racked up over the last three years, coupled with the ever-present possibility that she might need to jump on a plane at a moment's notice, there wasn't much room in the budget to travel for happy occasions. The airfare fund was for emergencies only.

Once we got through the preacher's theatrics, it was a quick "I do" and "I do too." Omar took a few pictures on his iPad. Aurélie's dress was from Forever 21 and cost $20. "If you have an eye, you can buy some stuff dere and you won't look like a simple tramp," she informed me.

The wedding took place one year to the day after she moved to New York. I was twenty-nine; she was twenty-eight. We didn't know it was day 365 until after the fact—or at least so she claims. When she noticed the coincidence, I told her she might have a *New York Times* bestseller on her hands: *How I Got My Green Card in 365 Days, and You Can Too!*

The proposal had been lackluster. During the weeks leading up to what would be our wedding day, we had conversation after conversation probing for a solution to the problem of it being illegal for her to stay in New York indefinitely. One day, standing in my bedroom, I just said, "Let's do it." She didn't look that pleased or convinced. "No, for real. Let's do it. I'll do it. You want to do it?"

"Yeah, fuck, I guess," she said.

"What else are we going to do? Not be together?"

"No."

"No, what?"

"No, we're not going to not be together. Ever."

The night before the wedding, we ate cheap ramen in the East Village and bought our wedding rings — $45 for the pair from a St. Marks incense store. The gentleman wanted $50. I set $45 cash on the table and asked him to kindly let me know before I crossed the threshold if I was shoplifting.

And so we were married. Joint tax return and everything. Aurélie could go to the doctor now and stay in the country. If we decided we didn't like each other so much after all, there would be paperwork to fill out, but we tried to tell ourselves that this hypothetical paperwork was the only thing that had changed. We were fake-real married. Fake because we didn't believe in it and real because I loved her so much that it felt like there was an actual energy field binding us together.

It wasn't only the Bird's two divorces that put me off the institution. The relationship between marriage and love had always struck me as tenuous at best, and Aurélie and I shared a deep revulsion of what marriage had become. Namely, bullshit. "You could feed all of Africa with da money people spend on weddings in a year," she said. "You have to spend all dat money so you can stand around and pretend to be a goddamn Disney princess for a day in a ridiculous costume dat you will never wear again, and all your friends are supposed to buy you a present. Fuck dat." But the United States of America insisted that I make an honest woman out of Aurélie or they'd send her packing back to Belgique. Couldn't have that.

In her accent, "I'm going to cook a bird" sounds like "I'm going to kooook a bird." She found the phrase amusing enough to repeat ad nauseam. "Kooook a bird. Kooook a big bird." Of course we didn't need a big bird; our first Thanksgiving together, the first Thursday after we got married, was in my Lower East Side apartment, just us. For two people who claimed to find marriage absurd, here we were, trying to create a Rockwellian experience.

Except nothing was going according to plan. I was not doing well. For weeks my arthritis had been making it difficult to sleep. I'd spent substantial portions of the prior three fall/winters in mental institutions, and aching joints, which flare up as soon as the first New York cold snap hits, had become an unwelcome reminder that madness season was upon us.

The wedding itself had caused some semi-sleepless nights. Even though she couldn't have been a better match for me if the Good Lord had crafted her out of my own rib, getting married was still a fairly seismic turn in how I'd seen my twenties shaking out.

Whirlwind romance aside, we had plenty to be stressed about. Due to her immigration status, Aurélie's work visa would expire at the end of the month. On my salary, there was no way we could afford our own place, so we were living with two roommates and would be doing so for the foreseeable future. Naturally, it wasn't much appreciated that she'd become a nonpaying fourth roommate, so in an effort to keep tensions low, we stayed out of the common area for the most part and she left every morning when I went to work, even if she had nowhere to go. She didn't dare leave a pink razor in the shower. We were, understandably enough, unwelcome guests in "our" home.

What little sleep I was getting came in weird intervals and at odd hours. I was desperate for every minute. Our whole schedule was dependent on when and for how long I could fall asleep. Add it all up, and it was enough to put mania in the starting blocks, waiting for the pistol.

So, on Thanksgiving, the roommates were gone and Aurélie *kooked* the bird by herself, taking breaks to come into the bedroom to rub my back while I tossed and turned and fought back tears. I hadn't fallen asleep until 7 a.m. the night before and was wide awake by 10. We ended up carving the turkey at midnight — I was napping at dinnertime, and even though she'd spent the whole day in the kitchen, she knew she couldn't wake me up. She put out quite the spread: sweet potatoes, green beans, mashed potatoes, turkey and gravy. *L'Amérique profonde* would have been proud. Our table was the ottoman in the middle of the living room. We both put on happy faces and snapped a couple of pics together — one of me carving the bird — but the smiles were pushed through gritted teeth.

By this point I knew my condition well. I knew the warning signs, I knew I had to deal with it at the first sign of trouble, and I knew what would happen and how quickly if I didn't. But knowledge is not prevention. In my case, knowledge only heightened my fear: the stakes were known. I'd done my best in the days leading up to Thanksgiving to work my medication and sleep regimen, but it didn't help that New York City did not give a shit about my bipolar disorder. The cold was indifferent to the arthritis it inflicted; 6 a.m. garbage trucks didn't care that I had been awake at 5:30 a.m.; the upstairs neighbors weren't about to inquire after my current sleep patterns before throwing a massive rager; and the fellas on the block still needed their Boricua music at the volume to which they were accustomed.

In a sure sign of trouble ahead, the most inconsequential nothings began to tie me in knots. Like Black Friday. Black fucking Friday. After we ate our bird and got into bed, I found myself staring at the ceiling, absolutely consumed with anxiety that I was going to blow my opportunity to buy the perfect pair of black leather Chelsea boots — "dancing shoes," I called them — at a substantial, once-a-year discount. We were throwing a not-a-wedding-reception party the following Saturday at my apartment, and I absolutely needed dancing shoes. Never mind the guest list was fifteen or so and the playlist would mostly consist of five-year-old indie rock tracks played at a reasonable volume.

These dancing shoes soon kicked off a Rube Goldberg–worthy anxiety sequence: *Isn't it okay to buy a little something for your own wedding party? Isn't it fucked that I, after not spending $100 combined on clothes within the last calendar year, am ready to throw myself out the window over boot angst? How much should I spend? Should we even have this goddamn party? My brother is coming to town — how high is he going to get? Should we get a photographer? Should we get a few? Can we get a DJ? Who do I know?! A DJ! Fuck, I hope my brother and I don't fight. We could have a red carpet! A fucking real bash! Fill the bathtub with champagne, and a trash barrel on the deck with cold beers! BBQ! Should we just cancel this thing? I'm not good. Can't cancel — what would we tell everyone?*

With all this pinging around in my head, I hardly slept. But I was jazzed the next morning anyway. A little dizzy, sure. And shaking a bit from sleep-deprived adrenaline and you-know-what's-around-the-corner-threat-level-yellow dread. My plan was to just get on with the day and go down for a nap as soon as I hit the wall. I didn't have to go to work and it was sweater weather outside — a perfect day to go tool around Manhattan with Aurélie. And get those boots.

Aurélie was *not* jazzed when I unfolded my Black Friday plan, but she wasn't about to turn me loose in SoHo alone. She wasn't blind to the fact that I'd been pissing money away like a Qatari prince; I couldn't go to the grocery store for a snack without dropping $100 on olives and cheese and cured meats. As I traipsed to the Ben Sherman dressing room, with no less than $500 in trousers and sweaters draped over my arm, Aurélie sank into the leather lounge chair, scowling. "Dancing shoes and you are rich now too? Dat's good news." I told her I wasn't getting it all and that I only owned one pair of jeans, and, yes, I *did* need a new coat.

Standing in the dressing room, staring at myself in the mirror, I suddenly felt a head rush that entered through my right ear and shook my brain around in my skull. The track lighting was swirling around me as if the roller-rink DJ had just announced, *All couples to the dance floor for the last skate of the night!* I had to urinate, and I found myself obsessing over one simple question: Why on God's green earth can't I just piss in the corner of this here booth? It seemed like a totally reasonable solution. How much different is it, really, than pissing in the woods? Both are technically illegal; neither prohibition is easy to enforce. I could just piss, march on out of here, and go home. I started unbuckling my pants, giggling a little as I slid them down. *I just don't give a fuck. Don't give a fuck about nothing,* I thought. *And everyone else does. All these fucking Black Friday sheep. What the fuck are we all doing here?*

I caught a look at my face in the mirror: wide, dilated pupils and big black circles. I'd seen that face before. It was the face of the guy who stays up all night making home music videos of himself dancing in a sombrero and covers the walls of his apartment in red Sharpie. He's supposed to have a Mohawk. His name is Myles. Myles ends up in the hospital.

Why can't you piss on the dressing room floor? Because it's fucking illegal. And because it's a dressing room floor. And because the floors are wood and it will run into the next stall, and because you don't do that. *You* don't do that. I had grabbed hold of my lucidity like a swinging vine and I needed to hold on. If there is a boundary line that separates Zack and Myles, I'd found it — toes hard against it. Piss over it and we're officially tits up.

I zipped my pants up and took off to find Aurélie. "I gotta go home — now," I told her. "I need a Risperdal." Then I dragged her to the register and rang it all up. She grabbed the receipt.

That night I alternated from bed to couch to porch and from cigs to deli meats to beer; all the while my brain refused to turn off: *How can people say that someone "belongs" in prison? How can a person "belong" in a societal construct? He's not a fish. Jail isn't water. He sure as shit won't die if he's not surrounded by iron bars. But what am I going to do to solve the prison–industrial complex? And what about third-world hunger? Why don't I work for UNICEF?*

To call the Bird or not to call the Bird? In those moments, that was always the question. *We'll talk too long… and I'm sick of waking her up at all hours. The woman needs her sleep too. And I'm a goddamn married man, a few months south of thirty.* I felt like a little boy, afraid of the dark, out of bed when he knows he shouldn't be.

Am I ever going to have a five-year plan or is my life going to be nothing more than a series of ad hoc attempts to stay sane? Should I just surrender? Buy the ticket and take the ride, go howl at the dark side of the moon for a while and see where I stand once I come out the other side?

I snuck into the bedroom and snapped about eighty-seven pictures of Aurélie sleeping that I intended to turn into a photo slideshow at the wedding party.

On Small Business Saturday, I woke up with a blazing sense of my own limitless creative potential. It had been well past dawn when I finally fell asleep, and as soon as I got out of bed two hours later, I absolutely had to write. I'd enrolled in a writing class that summer, and earlier that week the teacher had shown some interest in a piece she thought had potential to get published. It was called "A High-Class Hoops Feud at the Wichita Walmart," and it centered on how the Bird "about had to throw down" with a Walmart clerk because he made a smart-ass comment about her UVA Law sweatshirt. This was it, I was sure of it. Big break time. Get this thing published and soon agents would come calling. Book deal, maybe TV—who knows? I started a Twitter account just to put it on @NewYorker's radar—I liked my odds of making Shouts and Murmurs.

Aurélie and I had dinner plans, but that didn't matter to me. I was on the precipice. I insisted on working on the piece until almost 11 p.m., telling Aurélie, "Ten more minutes, I promise," the entire time. She'd hoped to have a calm meal, return to normalcy after all the Thanksgiving chaos, and finally spend some time together as newlyweds. But she'd thank me later, after this piece launched my career and we could finally afford our own place. As far as I was concerned, our pasta could wait.

On Cyber Monday, the dam broke. After submitting my piece, I spent all of Sunday and Monday afternoon obsessively checking my email, smoking, and waiting for editors to get back to me. *The New Yorker,* the *New York Times, McSweeney's*—they all had it in their inbox. I was not so far gone as to miss the parallels with my experience pre-Bellevue, and I knew that I was in bad shape. I could feel my brain burning white-hot, and if I squinted hard enough, I could see the molecules of solid objects start to bend—but fuck if I wasn't connecting dots in ways and at speeds that were so beautiful I could hardly stand it. I *did* have a teacher encouraging me, didn't I? She *did* give me the email addresses of her editor contacts, didn't she? It was all just enough to allow me to consider that the two realities could exist simultaneously: I could be both in the danger zone *and* on the verge of running down a dream.

When Aurélie came home from work, she found me on the floor in the fetal position, crying. I couldn't move; I'd gone out onto the terrace for a smoke a few hours earlier, looked down the thirty-foot drop to the concrete below, and realized I was too impaired to stand.

It wasn't that I had been thinking of jumping, but I was legitimately worried that I might think it would be fun to try to stand on the railing. Things were safer on the ground. From then on, I smoked in the apartment, stubbing out the butts in an empty Papa John's box.

I told her I couldn't get up. She said, "Den stay dere. You don't have to get up, monkey." She sat on my back and rubbed my head. "You don't have to worry because you're not going back to da hospital. You never go dere again. You don't belong dere." Then she cleaned the apartment, opened the windows, and lit some candles so it wouldn't smell like smoke when my roommates got home from work.

Even if you aren't a girl who's always dreamed of getting married, it's gotta be pretty shitty to have your husband go crazy a few days after your wedding. She did the best she could to keep a stiff upper lip, but watching me inch closer to the sheer drop of psychosis must have been terrifying. As the night wore on, it was clear to both of us that the poor girl was in over her head: reinforcements were needed.

So I called the Bird and handed the phone to my new bride. It's not the ideal way to meet your mother-in-law, but ideal goes out the window when the guy you just married is on the verge of a psychotic break. Aurélie unloaded the details of our saga thus far. To her surprise, the Bird said calmly, "I think he's okay." She told her that she was doing everything right and that she had to keep me straight on my meds. "Write it down. He forgets when he's tired." They made a plan to speak the next morning.

After another near sleepless night, I spent the better part of Giving Tuesday pacing the apartment, channeling first a wild and then a wounded animal. I tried to let the air out of the balloon on this writing bullshit. Who was I, to be expecting a personal email response from David Remnick within twenty-four hours? Hadn't I been surprised when the professor thought the thing was any good in the first place?

As soon as Aurélie got off work, Risperdal refills in hand, she came into the bedroom and told me she'd talked to my mom. The Bird had schooled her on the BP playbook. "Make a list with him of everything that's stressing him and then have him sort it into two categories: okay to worry about and not okay to worry about. Eliminate them one by one until his mind is calm enough to sleep." It was a tactic the Bird developed after my first break. Ever since, when I called her freaking out, instead of starting with "Calm down," she would just say, "Time to make a list, Gorilla?"

The Bird and I had been to hell and back together. Now it was Aurélie facing down the flames with me, sitting on the bed in this room I'd been pacing for hours. I took great comfort from the thought of her and the Bird, two powerhouses, working together, but I also felt horribly guilty for the burden I was putting on both of them, especially my new wife.

"Come on," she said, leaning forward to touch my hair, "make a list."

Z's List

1. I spent money on clothes, like an idiot. *Not okay to worry about. I have da receipt.*
2. I spent too much money on food and I can't get full. *Not okay to worry about. It's already in your belly. Order da $7.85 pad thai lunch special from da place on da corner. Quit eating olives.*
3. We don't have an apartment. We don't have any money. *Not okay to worry about today. We'll figure it out.*
4. I can't sleep. *You're going to sleep.*
5. I can't work. *Not okay to worry about. You're lucky to have a job dat understands. You won't get fired. Call your supervisor. Take da week off.*
6. Drugs aren't working. *Dey're going to work. Dey are working.*
7. I'm going to the hospital again. *No, you aren't. I won't let you.*
8. My back hurts. *I make you a bath.*

9. My arthritis hurts. *Take an ibuprofen.*

10. I'm dumb for writing. *What's done is done. Quit writing until you're back to normal.*

11. It's happening. It's always going to keep happening. *It's not always going to happen. It's getting better.*

12. You don't deserve this. You shouldn't have to do this. *Dat's nonsense. I do anything for you.*

Once Aurélie fell asleep, I snuck into the bathroom and called the Bird myself. Making the list with Aurélie had calmed me down, but I needed more reassurance. When she heard my voice, she said, "You sound like an old arthritic gorilla with patches of fur missing on his back." I read her my list. "You got this," she told me. "That girl loves and understands you. Not the easiest combination to come by. I know you're safe with her."

"Why do I keep having to deal with this? I really wish this wasn't happening again."

"Boy, as Pa always says, 'You can wish in one hand and shit in the other.' You got the BP."

"This isn't my fault," I told the Bird.

"It's not."

I started crying, hard. Of course intellectually I could latch on to the idea that I didn't choose to be mentally ill. I could parrot my own bullshit about how no one chooses to be sick and about how the mentally ill are no different from diabetics or cancer patients, but did I really believe me?

Sniveling and watching myself ugly-cry in the bathroom mirror, I laughed in my own face. I could either accept that I was suffering from random chance, a bad bounce, or continue to say these things about "random chance" out loud while privately considering myself a defective piece of shit.

"No, but really," I told the Bird, "it's not my fault."

"It's not, baby. It's really, really, really not." I could hear her heart breaking for me.

I left the bathroom, made a cup of tea, popped another Risperdal, and recorded it in my little black medication notebook. Underneath *2 mg Risperdal 1:07 a.m.,* I wrote *I am okay. I will be okay. This is hard. Hard is okay. I am not going crazy.*

I checked in on Aurélie: she was out cold. The week's events had pushed her to the brink of her own sanity and that's only a slight exaggeration. She was worn-out from staying up with me, worn-out from me snapping at her for suggesting that spending $100 on fancy snacks was unsustainable, worn-out from worrying that I wouldn't be okay. She looked so serene there in the bed, clutching her filthy old one-eyed stuffed blue dog that she'd had since she was a little girl. Watching her sleep, I thought: if she had gone to one of the other thousands of bars on the Lower East Side of Manhattan that night, if I'd left the bar twenty minutes earlier, if NYU MBA students didn't like talking about their accomplishments so much, if, if, if…I didn't want to wake her, so I grabbed a pillow and headed to the living room.

The solution to mania is so simple yet so hard to come by. Just sleep.

The couch can be a nice refuge from the insomniac's bed—a little less pressure. I put a little DVR'd English Premier League on the TV and let that beautiful grass and those calming witty Brits rock me back and forth at low volume. I used the game clock to track how long I'd been on my back, heavy eyelids but still conscious: seventeenth minute, thirty-third, forty-sixth, halftime. I focused on my breathing while the talking heads praised an overmatched West Ham's grit against a loaded Manchester City squad.

I still wasn't asleep when the ref pointed to the center circle and whistled for the second half to start, so I tried a relaxation technique I'd read about: I started with my toes and imagined them filling up with sand. Only after the toes were completely full did I move on to my feet, then ankles, shins, thighs, waist. I prayed to be knocked out before I got to my torso, but every time I started to slip into something resembling sleep, my brain would catch on a dying ember of thought and roar back to life.

Next, I imagined giant humpback whales gliding through the ocean, and I tried to become a whale myself—all fat and heavy, with those big ol' eyelids slowly closing.

Finally, some combination of modern pharmacology, the Barclays English Premier League, sand in my toes, and the eyelids of great whales put me down. It wasn't the most restful sleep I'd ever experienced, but when I opened my eyes, the sun was streaming into the living room and I had no recollection of the prior five hours. I was up before Aurélie and chipper when she woke. This did not please her.

"Did you sleep at all? Why are you up? Should you get back in bed?"

I told her that we'd landed a clean body shot to the BP. The twister was still visible but it was retreating into the distance. Sure, the lawn was fucked-up and a few windowpanes were shattered, but the roof was still attached and the car was in the driveway. "Let's get food. I'm starving."

We took a walk through the East Village. On the way to our local coffee shop, we sidestepped no fewer than five severely mentally ill homeless people and we did exactly what everyone else around us did: ignored them. The level of need-blindness required to get an omelet in New York City is staggering; you'd starve if you stopped at every emergency in your sight line.

"I think I made it," I said. "I don't feel great, but I feel safe. I feel like myself."

She looked unconvinced.

"Are you mad?" I asked.

"No, just stressed."

"It's okay if you are."

"I know."

"I wish I could promise that this will never happen again. I'm sorry."

"Don't need to tell me you're sorry. It's not your fault you get sick. I'm happy you feel better, but it's been shit for so long dat my brain can't catch up. I never seen dat before. It broke my heart. And I never want to cry in front of you because you were so stressed, so I've been crying in da bathroom at work every day and trying to pretend everything is all right. I don't sleep neither. I feel like I been to da war."

After breakfast, we grabbed a couple fancy lattes we couldn't afford and sat on a bench in Tompkins Square Park, where three years earlier I'd galloped like a dog and nearly shot a round of H-O-R-S-E with Daniel Day-Lewis. Aurélie squeezed my biceps and rested her head on my shoulder. She seemed to be finally entertaining the possibility that her baptism by fire had ended, that maybe it was safe to exhale. We both just shut up for a while and took in the pigeons and the chess players and the marvelous number of seemingly unemployed New Yorkers who somehow had enough money to wander around the park in $1,000 Moncler jackets on a Wednesday afternoon. Of course there were an equal number of homeless people dragging shopping-cart jalopies with bungee-corded milk crates holding all of their worldly possessions. Luck of the draw.

I knew we'd never have kids—not with the radioactive nature of my genetic material; I'd never risk passing this on. I also knew I could never withstand what the Bird had gone through with me in the psych ward; I'd rather be patient than parent any day. But maybe one day a sleepless night wouldn't leave me terrified by the brittle nature of my own lucidity.

After what felt like ten minutes of silence, Aurélie looked up at me with those big brown fearless eyes. "I teach you some French: *Je suis un gorille bipolaire.*"

I am a bipolar gorilla.

Acknowledgments

Bird, Granny and Pa (miss you). Adam and Corryn, Alexa, Pete, and little Ellie. King Edward, Lala and Amelia. Grandad.

Mike and Sarah Keenan, Elliott Klass, Andrew Kewley, Kent Russell, Eve Mattucci, Jerry Portwood, Bryan Sipe, Doug Bouton, Amy FitzHenry. Bobby Prince Jr., James Tichenor. Ryan Boyle and Ari Moore, Omar Agha-Kahala, Sian-Pierre and Joe Regis, Justin Milner, Mike Patton, Rob Lindsey and Colleen Herman. The Heyman Bros. Dr. Al, Rashad H., Mark Hitchcock, Jon Miller, Josh Grubaugh, Alec Zadek, Natalie Blazer, Jason Watson, Tom Slaughter, Jonas Jacobson. Jayson Haedrich and Amanda Hamann; Scott Ruplinger; Chele Behrens; Rob Howes; Lance, Bob, and Jana Hublick; Lisa Smith; Matthew and Michael Stewart. Kathryn Liverani, Matt Berman, Jacob Rolls, Greg Gomez. Chico "Hapa" Herbison, Professor Brendan Garrett, Dean Goluboff, and Dean Jeffries: "He was on the boat!" Coach Bribiesca, Jared Rhodes, Preston Brin, Desmond Johnson. Kiese Laymon, Carla Eckels, Sean Cole, Ira Glass. Kenny and Keith Lucas, Gad Elmaleh.

The Legal Aid Society of New York.

Jon Bliss, Dr. Singh.

Jason Richman and Mary Pender at UTA. Andrew Schneider, Peter Kiernan, and Free Association.

Malin von Euler-Hogan, Reagan Arthur, Judy Clain, Craig Young, Lauren Velasquez, Julie Ertl, Lena Little, Sabrina Callahan, and Karen Landry at Little, Brown.

Acknowledgments

Jean Garnett, my brilliant editor and amigo.

Farley Chase, my agent, my friend. Away we go.

"Aurélie's Friend" Rachel Lovell.

Nicole Hagen.

Aurélie, my love, my Porg.

About the Author

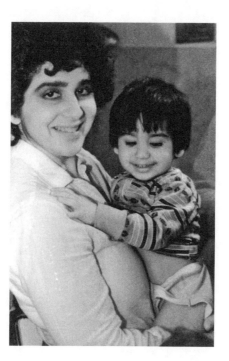

Zack McDermott has worked as a public defender for the Legal Aid Society of New York. His work has appeared on *This American Life*, *Morning Edition*, and *Gawker*, among other places. He lives in Brooklyn and Los Angeles.